SCREENING CHILDREN FOR BRAIN IMPAIRMENT

Richard Berg, Ph.D., was trained in clinical neuropsychology at the University of Houston and completed a postdoctoral fellowship in neuropsychology at the University of Nebraska Medical Center. Dr. Berg formerly worked at the St. Jude Children's Research Hospital in Memphis and currently directs the neuropsychology laboratory for the West Virginia University Medical Center in Charleston.

Michael Franzen, Ph.D., was trained in clinical psychology at Southern Illinois University and completed a clinical internship and a postdoctoral year of training in clinical neuropsychology at the University of Nebraska Medical Center. Dr. Franzen is currently Director of Neuropsychology for the West Virginia University School of Medicine in Morgantown and he serves as Director of Psychological Training and Research at Allegheny General Hospital in Pittsburgh.

Both of the authors have published widely in the field of clinical neuropsychology and are actively involved in ongoing research.

SCREENING CHILDREN FOR BRAIN IMPAIRMENT

Michael Franzen, Ph.D.
Richard Berg, Ph.D.

Alliant International University
Los Angeles Campus Library
1000 South Fremont Ave., Unit 5
Alhambra, CA 91803

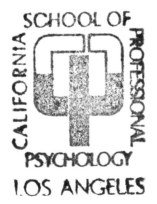

SPRINGER PUBLISHING COMPANY
New York

Copyright © 1989 by Springer Publishing Company, Inc.

All rights reserved

No part of this publication may be reproduced, stored in a retrieval system, or transmitted in any form or by any means, electronic, mechanical, photocopying, recording, or otherwise, without the prior permission of Springer Publishing Company, Inc.

Springer Publishing Company, Inc.
536 Broadway
New York, NY 10012

89 90 91 92 93 / 5 4 3 2 1

Library or Congress Cataloging-in-Publication Data

Franzen, Michael D., 1954–
    Screening Children for brain impairment.

    Bibliography: p.
    Includes index.
    1. Brain damage—Diagnosis. 2. Brain—damaged children—Medical examinations. 3. Pediatric neurology.
I. Berg, Richard (Richard A.) II. Title.
RJ496.B7F73   1989   618.92'80475   88-32742
ISBN 0-8261-6390-4

Printed in the United States of America

Contents

Introduction	ix
Part I Cerebral Disorders in Children and the Specialists Who Treat Them	1
1 The Differing Roles of Professional Specialties	3
Pediatrician	5
Behavioral Pediatrician	6
Pediatric Neurologist	6
Child Psychiatrist	7
Child Neuropsychologist	7
School Psychologist	8
Relationship Between Results of Neuropsychological and Achievement Assessment	8
Overview	11
2 Developmental Disorders	12
Mental Retardation	13
Genetic Disorders	15
Exposure to Neurotoxins	17
Vitamin and Other Nutritional Deficiencies	18
Sensory Disorders	20
Auditory Disorders	21
Language Disorders	21
Overview	22
3 Neurological Disorders of Childhood	23
Seizure Disorders	23

Hydrocephalus 26
Tourette Syndrome 27
Muscular Dystrophies 28
Other Disorders of Neuromuscular Development 29
Cerebral Palsy 30
Head Injury 30
Overview 32

4 Psychiatric and Behavioral Disorders of Children 33
Conduct Disorders 34
Childhood Schizophrenia 34
Affective Disorders 34
Anxiety Disorders 35
Eating Disorders 35
Infantile Autism 35
Attention Deficit Disorder 36
Developmental Motor Disorders 37
Learning Disorders 37
Disorders Not Otherwise Specified (NOS) 38

5 Neurological Soft Signs 39
The Controversy Related to Soft Signs 40
Relationship of Soft Signs to Neurological Disorders 41
Disorders Associated with Soft Signs 42
Classification and Assessment of Soft Signs 43
Neurological Dysfunction of Children (NDOC) 48
Physical and Neurological Examination for Soft Signs 49
Overview 50

Part II Evaluating the Child 51

6 The Interview and History 53
Interviewing the Child 53
Interviewing the Parents 58
Interviewing School Personnel 59
Obtaining the History 60
Conclusions 68

7 The Mental Status Exam in Children 70
Essentials of the Extended Mental Status Exam for Children 72
Attention 73
Language 74
Memory 77
Constructional Abilities 78
Higher Cognitive Functions 79
Summary 79

Contents

8 The Wechsler Intelligence Scale for Children-Revised as a Screening Device   80
- WISC-R Verbal-Performance Discrepancies   81
- Wechsler Subtests as Screening Devices   83
- Effects of Brain Dysfunction on WISC-R Performance   86

9 The Kaufman Assessment Battery for Children   90
- Theoretical Basis of the K-ABC   90
- The K-ABC Subtests   92
- The K-ABC as a Screening Instrument for Brain Dysfunction   99

Part III   Assessment Instruments and Their Uses   101

10 Screening Tests for Perceptual, Cognitive, and Motor Functioning   103
- Visual Functions   105
- Visual Recognition   106
- Complex Visual Functions   108
- Auditory Functions   118
- Tactile Functions   121
- General Cognitive Functions   124
- Manual Motor Functioning   129

11 Verbal Screening Instruments   133
- "Normal" Language Development   134
- Language Disorders in Children   135
- Childhood Aphasia   136
- Tests for Aphasia   138
- Screening for Verbal Fluency   148
- Academic Skills   150

12 Screening Children for Memory Functions   154
- Verbal Memory and Learning Problems   155
- Visual Memory Functioning   162
- Tactile Memory—The Tactual Performance Test   171

Part IV   Special Considerations in Assessment   175

13 Screening Batteries for Children   177
- Screening Batteries versus Single Tests versus Comprehensive Test Batteries   177
- Wysocki and Sweet Screening Battery   181
- Florida Kindergarten Screening Battery   184
- The McCarthy Screening Test   185
- Screening Test for the Luria–Nebraska Neuropsychological Battery   186
- The Clinical Neuropsychological Evaluation Instrument   187
- Discriminant Equation for Screening for Neuropsychological Abnormality   188

14 Assessment of Very Young Children 190
General Screening Devices of Cognitive Abilities 191
Screening for Social and Adaptive Behavior 196

Appendices
Appendix A Sample Interview Form 203
Appendix B Common Tests Used in the Assessment of School-Aged Children 208
Appendix C Common Tests Used in the Assessment of Preschool-Aged Children 211
Appendix D Test Publisher Addresses 213

Glossary 215

References 227

Index 239

Introduction

This book arose partly out of the response to our earlier book *Screening for Brain Impairment* (Berg, Franzen, & Wedding; 1987). That book attempted to provide general clinicians working with an adult population with the basic knowledge to recognize and screen for the presence of organic etiologies. We decided to limit the information to adult disorders in order to maintain a reasonable length for the book. The response to that book has been gratifying and has influenced the decision to write the present one.

This book is intended for the general clinician who sees children as part of his/her professional practice. Often in the course of general practice, the psychologist or physician is asked to evaluate a child and determine whether or not an organic impairment is responsible for particular behavioral manifestations. Due to the limitations of training or experience, the general child clinician cannot be expected to provide a specialized assessment. However, they are still faced with the question of when to refer for a more extensive specialized evaluation which can be expensive in terms of time and money. This book is not meant to teach specialized evaluation; only years of didactic and experiential training can do that. But this book can be helpful in learning to perform an initial evaluation that can answer the question of whether to refer.

General child clinicians have already received specialized training in the area of child or pediatric practice. Optimally, this has included training in developmental theory. Just as this training sets them apart from adult general clinicians, so have child neuropsychologists received training that sets them apart from adult neuropsychologists. It is to a child neuropsychologist (or pediatrician, child psychiatrist, or pediatric neurologist as described in the first chapter of this book) that the child patient should be referred.

In an ideal world, the child patient has equal access to a wide variety of specialists. In the real world, access is limited due to geography and the limited amount of training experiences and institutions available to the professional seeking to become a specialist. Therefore, access to a specialist often involves extra effort and time as well as the additional distance required. Another consideration is the fact that parents or school teachers usually do not have the acumen required to recognize organic etiologies resulting in the referral of children with central nervous system etiologies to general child clinicians. They, then, must be able to recognize the possibility of an organic etiology and refer accordingly.

To evaluate the possibility of organic etiologies, it is necessary for child clinicians to utilize procedures that may not have been taught to them during their training. A major purpose of this book is to describe those procedures that can be employed without the additional specialized training of a child clinical neuropsychologist. Most of the procedures and tests described in this book can be acquired and used without a large monetary investment. Another purpose of this book is to educate the general child clinician as to the various type of disorders and their clinical presentations. A third purpose is to demystify the language and procedures of the child clinical neuropsychologist to further communication between the generalist and the specialist, thereby favorably effecting the overall level of patient care. For that reason, we have included a glossary of common technical terms. Finally, our experience with referring clinicians as well as our experience in developing curriculum and providing graduate education has indicated that most training programs do not currently provide adequate training in techniques to recognize and evaluate neuropsychological disorders. We hope that this book will be used in the training of future child clinicians to remediate that unfortunate but understandable problem.

We will not cover developmental aspects of behavioral and cognitive growth and change in this book. This is a very complex topic, and we do not feel we can do justice to the topic in the limited span of this book. By not discussing developmental theory, we do not mean to imply that it is unimportant. It is essential that every clinician who sees children has a working knowledge of developmental theory. In addition, the clinician should have knowledge of neurological developmental theory. There are many texts available, several of which are excellent. We would recommend Illington (1980, 1982). Failure to meet milestones at the usual time does not necessarily mean that the child is neurologically impaired, but it does raise the likelihood that a more complete evaluation might be in order.

Not every patient should receive every procedure described in this book. However, by studying this book the clinician can develop an outline for a

Introduction

child evaluation that seeks to uncover organic etiologies and aid in the decision to refer. The first step is to obtain as complete a history as is possible. The history may help to uncover organic etiologies as well as provide useful information to the specialist when the referral is made. If the history uncovers the possibility of an organic etiology, that particular problem area should receive special attention during the second step of the evaluation, the mental status exam. Finally, if the clinician judges herself to be competent in the use of the screening tests described in this book, those procedures can be administered in a further evaluation of the problem area. In no case are the procedures described in this book intended to take the place of an extensive specialized evaluation.

There are three possible outcomes of the extended mental status exam described in this book. First the evaluation may result in no indication of an organic etiology, in which case no referral is made. (Of course if there is any doubt, further evaluation is necessary to rule out the possibility.) Second, the mental status exam may result in a suspicion that organic impairment is present, in which case the child clinician performs one of the techniques described in the chapters on screening tests. This will allow greater specification of the type and degree of impairment present. Third, there may be sufficient evidence from the history and mental status exam to justify referral to a specialist.

In addition to the information contained in this book, clinicians can obtain information from the specialists to whom they may refer a patient. In general, we recommend that a consumer-oriented attitude be adopted by the clinician. Contact the specialist by telephone and describe the problem, asking for advice about whether a referral is warranted. Following referral and receipt of a report from the specialist, the generalist can again contact the specialist to ask for clarification and to give feedback about the usefulness of the report. Specialists tend to use jargon, and additional communication can avoid misunderstandings. Finally, the generalist can seek out a specialist with whom she feels comfortable and with whom a good pattern of communication can be developed. The specialist can provide feedback about the degree of specificity desired in the referral question, further increasing the quality of communication.

OVERVIEW OF THE BOOK

It would be impossible to contain in a single book all of the information necessary to evaluate a child and to screen for the possibility of organic involvement in the factors responsible for the child's behavior. It is even more apparent that it would be impossible to communicate the skills necessary to such an evaluation via the printed word. We therefore hope that clinicians and students who use this book will supplement it with additional readings and with supervised clinical experience. However, we feel that the information contained in this book cannot be found in a single source elsewhere. As mentioned earlier, in this book, we assume that the reader is familiar with the basics of child developmental theory, especially as it pertains to neurological and psychological aspects of development. We also assume that the reader is familiar with psychological assessment and with the clinical method.

The book opens with a discussion of the various roles of the different professionals who have chosen to evaluate and treat children. We hope this information will provide a basis for enhanced interdisciplinary communication and encourage each to use the other's skills to the benefit of the child patient.

The next section of the book gives an overview of some of the most commonly seen neurological and psychiatric/behavioral disorders in children. This serves to alert clinicians to the types of disorders seen and the common presentations of these disorders. Of course before treating children with these problems, more information is needed.

The following section presents aspects of the evaluation of the child that can be conducted without any special equipment and with the skills already in the possession of adequately trained child clinicians. These evaluative instruments are the interview, history, mental status exam, and the evaluation for soft neurological signs. Although most adequately trained child clinicians should be able to use these instruments, and may in fact be already using them, it will take a slightly different focus to implement the instruments as screening devices for organic impairment. The clinician can be guided here by the material in this book and by other knowledge obtained from the current literature and neuropsychologically oriented texts.

The next section contains several chapters devoted to specific assessment instruments. Some, such as the Wechsler Intelligence Scale for Children-Revised, are quite well known to most child clinicians. Others such as the Kaufman Assessment Battery for Children may be novel to the general child clinician because of their relatively recent appearance. Still other instruments, such as the Rey Auditory Verbal Learning Test, may be unfamiliar to the general child clinician because it has previously been used mainly in specialized settings.

The final two chapters are on topics that are not easily categorized with the previous chapters. There is a chapter devoted to a discussion of various screening batteries for children that have been suggested in the literature. The other chapter is a discussion of issues related to the evaluation of the very young child. Finally, the Appendices contain a sample interview form that readers can adopt and change to suit their own clinical settings and

Introduction

populations, a list of tests commonly used to evaluate school-aged children, a list of tests commonly used to evaluate preschool-aged children, and a list of test publisher addresses.

We hope that this book will be useful to the practicing general child clinician. We also hope that it will be useful to the graduate student. Both groups of people can use the book to increase their knowledge of cortical dysfunction and to increase their repertoire of clinical assessment techniques. Our ultimate hope is that the use of this book will help increase the standard of care for patients.

SCREENING CHILDREN FOR BRAIN IMPAIRMENT

Part I
CEREBRAL DISORDERS IN CHILDREN AND THE SPECIALISTS WHO TREAT THEM

1
The Differing Roles of Professional Specialists

The disorders and screening procedures discussed in this book can lead to referral of patients to a range of specialists. Before exploring the question of when to refer, it is useful to have a clear picture of the roles of various specialists who treat children with behavioral problems or suspected neurological disorders. Although there is some overlap and apparent similarities among the different speciality areas, it is important to take into account the different emphases in training and in the approach to a problem. For example, both a behavioral pediatrician and a child neuropsychologist might ask a child to draw a circle. However, the scoring systems used by the two professionals would be different, as would the uses to which the derived information is put. So, although the functions of a pediatrician, a child psychiatrist, a behavioral pediatrician, a pediatric neurologist, and a child neuropsychologist may appear similar, the general clinician would not want to refer to one when it would be more appropriate to refer to another.

The generalist who is faced with making a referral to a specialist may therefore find herself in somewhat of a quandary. To whom can the generalist refer? Part of the answer lies in knowing something about the different specialties and this chapter will briefly review each of them. First, however, we will explore another aspect of knowing to whom to refer. It involves developing relationships with specialists in the local professional community. This is an important context for patient care.

For those clinicians who live in communities with teaching hospitals, developing relationships is somewhat easier at first. By consulting the listing of professionals at a teaching hospital, one can at least find out if specialists with the requisite training are available at that particular site. However, the presence of a teaching hospital does not remove the generalist's responsibility to develop relationships with specialists.

The general clinician should adopt a consumer-oriented attitude when choosing a specialist. The general child clinician can ask for a copy of the curriculum vitae of the specialist and can also ask about the licensure and possible board certification. Although the ultimate consumer of the specialist's services is the patient, the clinician is in a better position to evaluate the utility of the information and services obtained from the specialist. Since the generalist is also partly a consumer of the specialist's information, he should evaluate whether the information derived from the report of the specialist is useful in completing the assessment and determining the treatment of the patient.

The language of specialists differs from the language of generalists. The specific vocabulary (or jargon) of different specialists also differs among themselves. The generalist can help ensure that the specialist is providing useful information by inquiring about the meaning of terms with which she is unfamiliar. Specialists, just like other humans, sometimes assume too much about the ability of the other person to understand what is being communicated. The generalist should not assume that the familiar meaning of the term is the intended meaning. For example, short-term memory has very different meanings for psychologists and physicians. Communication between professions should be descriptively behavior-oriented to help obviate any misunderstandings. For example, instead of saying that the child showed deficits in short-term memory, the clinician can say that the child could remember only three of five words following a five-minute delay.

Just as the specialist has a responsibility to use nonjargon language in communicating with the nonspecialist, the generalist has a responsibility to learn some of the basic terms in the specialist's lexicon. Generalists should be very careful about using these terms in their own communication. As noted above, the general clinician should always ask the meaning of terms that may be open to various interpretations.

When making a referral to a specialist, it is wise to remember the golden rule, namely, do unto others as you would have them do unto you. Just as a general clinician likes to receive as much information as possible before seeing a patient, so does the specialist. This information can consist of copies of pertinent medical records, school records, and evaluations based on the general clinician's examination. The general clinician should state the results of any screening procedures that were performed. The results should be presented in the form of a description of performance rather than as an interpretation. The information can be given to the parents in a sealed envelope, but it is preferable to send the information through the mail as far in advance of the appointment as possible.

The referral question should be as specific as possible. Examples include, "Is there an organic etiology to the temper tantrums?", "Are the problems in sustained attention amenable to medical intervention?", or "What are the implications of the child's head injury for academic achievement, and is a special educational intervention likely to be helpful?", rather than "Please evaluate this child."

Part of developing a relationship with a specialist is providing feedback to the specialist about the relative utility of the report. Telephone contact following the receipt of the report can help clarify any ambiguous points as well as address those that may not have been included in the original referral but were raised by the content of the report.

The need for a continuing relationship is also based on the concept of continuity of care. In most cases, the specialist will not follow the child over the course of his development; that is the role of the generalist. Referring the patient to the same specialist for a follow-up evaluation will help increase the reliability of the information. Continued contact with a specialist can help educate the general clinician in terms of what to expect from a specialist as well as sensitize the general clinician regarding which signs to look for in a patient.

There are probably as many specialists as there are child problems. However, the child clinician is likely to come into contact with a pediatrician, a behavioral pediatrician, a pediatric neurologist, a child psychiatrist, a child neuropsychologist, or a school psychologist.

PEDIATRICIAN

A pediatrician is a physician who limits her practice to the treatment of children. Similar to a family doctor, a pediatrician will follow a child throughout growth, often treating him or her well into adolescence. The pediatrician receives the normal physician's training consisting of four years of medical school and an internship. In addition, the pediatrician will usually complete a residency in pediatrics; in fact this residency is required for board certification. The pediatric residency will often include rotations in family practice, neurology, and medicine. Other rotations may include psychiatry and surgery. Most parents are referred to a pediatrician by the obstetrician who provided prenatal care to the mother and subsequently delivered the baby. The pediatrician will usually have all of the medical records for the child including the history, schedule of immunizations, and treatment for any of the childhood diseases. Because pediatricians provide treatment for illnesses as well as routine examinations over a period of time, they can be excellent sources of information regarding the medical history of the child.

BEHAVIORAL PEDIATRICIAN

Behavioral pediatricians are physicians who specialize in the assessment and treatment of childhood diseases. They usually have a strong foundation in developmental theory. They differ from other pediatricians in that their assessments often involve evaluation of behavioral aspects of development. Behavioral pediatricians are more likely to include aspects of the child–parent interaction in their evaluations. Most pediatricians will also include the interaction as part of the evaluation, but the behavioral pediatrician will place a greater emphasis on the interaction. Other components of the behavioral pediatrician's evaluation include the physician–child interaction and performance of the child on various developmental tasks, such as informal assessments of drawing, language use, and motor skills. The behavioral pediatrician is also likely to have performed an elementary form of a neurological evaluation.

PEDIATRIC NEUROLOGIST

A pediatric neurologist is a physician who has completed the usual medical training and a residency in neurology. Many pediatric neurologists subsequently complete a fellowship in pediatric neurology. These physicians specialize in neurological disorders of childhood, which include abnormalities of the central nervous system and peripheral nervous system. Their evaluations include a general physical examination which is then supplemented by a detailed neurological evaluation. Here, emphasis is placed on the presence of abnormal reflexes, the development of motor skills and strength, and the development of cognitive skills. If a child has a neurological disorder such as epilepsy, a pediatric neurologist may be following the treatment of the child. However, it is more likely that a pediatric neurologist has a child referred to him for evaluation; the medical follow-up then is provided by the child's pediatrician or family physician. Other problems for which a pediatric neurologist may have received a referral include headaches, delayed motor or cognitive development, and specific neuromuscular disorders.

The child with a diagnosis of cerebral palsy requires special consideration. As a diagnosis, "cerebral palsy" is not informative. The term is used as a description of any child who has received an injury or insult to the central nervous system as a result of prenatal or perinatal factors or factors related to the delivery process. Because the term "cerebral palsy" is nonspecific for type of etiology or presentation, it is important to obtain records specifying the type of injury and the course of the sequelae. The records of a pediatric neurologist can be very helpful in this regard because they are likely to contain an outline of the developmental milestones.

CHILD PSYCHIATRIST

A child psychiatrist receives the usual medical training of a physician, but the elective rotations are more likely to be in family medicine and pediatrics. Following residency, a fellowship in child psychiatry is often completed. Here the emphasis in training is on the identification and treatment of childhood behavioral disorders. Depending on the training program, the child psychiatrist may receive training in both medical treatment and in psychological treatment modalities. Evaluations include review of the results of the physical examinations (or performing one if one has not been done), assessment of the child–parent interactions, and conducting a mental status exam of the child. Many child psychiatrists work with child psychologists who perform psychological testing of the child.

Although child psychiatrists may function as a referred specialist, they are likely to follow a child if a treatable psychiatric disorder has been diagnosed. Therefore, the records of the child psychiatrist or a conversation with the child psychiatrist can provide much useful information to the general clinician. The child psychiatrist is likely to have information related to child development, the parent–child interaction dynamics, peer relationships of the child, and personality development. Problems for which a child psychiatrist may treat a child include recurrent bedwetting, emotional difficulties, attention deficit disorder (which may also be seen by pediatricians), and conduct disorders.

CHILD NEUROPSYCHOLOGIST

The child neuropsychologist is a psychologist who has received specialized training in neuropsychology and then specialized in the assessment of children. Child neuropsychologists optimally receive training in developmental theory, child psychopathology, and human developmental neurobiology. Although there are no legal or formal standards for designating a person as a child neuropsychologist, these individuals usually receive graduate training in clinical psychology, followed by an internship that allows them to concentrate in clinical neuropsychology. The child neuropsychologist will preferably complete a postdoctoral fellowship specifically in child neuropsychology. Often the training in neurological theory and developmental neurobiology is obtained in the form of seminars during the postdoctoral year.

Although many child neuropsychologists, especially recently trained ones, may treat children for developmental disorders, or acquired problems such as those subsequent to head injury, most child neuropsychologists are likely to see a child for a referred evaluation. The identified problem at the time of referral may include recent changes in behavior or affective functioning that are resistant to psychological or medical means of treatment, difficulty in academic performance, or some event such as a seizure disorder or a head injury.

The evaluation conducted by a child clinical neuropsychologist includes assessment of the parent–child interaction, a complete history, intellectual assessment, review of school records, the use of specific neuropsychological instruments, and evaluation of behavioral and emotional functioning. Frequently, the child clinical neuropsychologist will include some standardized measures of achievement in his evaluation.

SCHOOL PSYCHOLOGIST

At present, the professional role of the school psychologist is in the midst of redefinition. Originally, the school psychologist served as a counselor who had training in the administration and interpretation of tests of intellectual functioning and academic achievement. Recent years have witnessed an expansion of the role of the school psychologist to include evaluation of personality functioning and some forms of neuropsychological assessment. There is at least one training program in school psychology (Ball State University) that allows the student to specialize in neuropsychological assessment of the child. Usually the focus of neuropsychological assessment conducted by a school psychologist is centered around those aspects of neuropsychological functioning that impact on academic achievement. That is one difference from the child clinical neuropsychologist, who in addition focuses on the aspects of neuropsychological functioning that may be related to medical or psychiatric diagnosis. Although most school psychologists work for a board of education in a school setting, some are now working in private practice.

RELATIONSHIP BETWEEN RESULTS OF NEUROPSYCHOLOGICAL AND ACHIEVEMENT ASSESSMENT

In one sense, it can be said that the central job of the child is to learn. This learning occurs both in school and in less structured settings. The evaluation of learning that occurs outside of the school setting is less formal. Although this learning may be no less important to the overall functioning of the child, it is less frequently the reason for a referral to a health care provider. On the other hand, suspicion of academic achievement difficulties is often a reason for referral to a wide variety of professionals including family practitioners, pediatricians, neurologists, psychiatrists, and clinical psychologists. One helpful source of background information is the report card. Unfortunately, there is great variability in the meaning of grades across both school systems and teachers. A more reliable form of information can be derived from the results of standardized academic achievement testing.

The results of standardized academic achievement testing have the advantage of being comparable across time and setting. For example, it may be difficult to interpret a grade of "A" given to a fifth grade special education class. The "A" may be related more to the teacher's perception of effort expended by the child than to the level of skill demonstrated by the child in the topic area. However, a standard score of 35th percentile on a standardized test of reading skill is interpretable as reading at a level superior to 35% of the children of the same age tested in the normative sample.

Many standardized tests of academic achievement provide for the transformation of scores to grade equivalencies. Although these grade equivalents may have the seductive property of seeming to be readily interpretable, there are many problems attendant in their use. For example, most children "lose" a little academic achievement over the summer break. But for the equivalency scores, a result of fifth grade–first month is always higher than fourth grade–ninth month. In addition, the scale characteristics of grade equivalencies are often unknown, resulting in difficulties in interpreting any changes. The same problems are present, although to a lesser extent, in age-equivalent scores. It is preferable to report and interpret raw scores and standard scores, possibly presented in the form of percentiles or in standardized scores based on the distribution in the normative or reference sample such as T-scores or Z-scores.

In some instances, the academic achievement testing of the child may be conducted by a child neuropsychologist. In some instances the neuropsychological evaluation of a child may be conducted by a school psychologist. In either case, the optimal situation involves the combination of the information into a reasonable set of conclusions, tempered by the history, the assessment of personality functioning, and the behavioral observations.

The difference between neuropsychologial and achievement evaluation instruments helps to place the interaction between the two in high relief. Neuropsychological assessment instruments are usually aimed at evaluating a cortico-behavioral function. That function may play a role in academic achievement, but it is not interchangeable with academic achievement. For example, as part of a neuropsychological evaluation a psychologist may administer a test of attention. Attention certainly plays a large role in academic achievement; however, once we have determined that the child is capable of adequate attention, we would not assume that the child had used her attentional skills to achieve at an age-appropriate level. Her achievement is also a function of her motivation, her emotional well-being, and the skill of the teachers.

In addition, neuropsychological assessment instruments usually promote the evaluation of optimal functioning by instructing the administrator to test the limits and question any ambiguities. On the other hand, the achievement instruments are aimed at evaluating the usual level of functioning of the child. Some of these tests can be administered in a group format, lessening the likelihood that testing the limits or further evaluating any ambiguous answers can occur.

The use of tests of intellectual functioning occurs in both academic and neuropsychological settings. For example, the Wechsler Intelligence for Children-Revised (WISC-R) is an almost ubiquitous instrument. However, the school psychologist and the neuropsychologist put the results of the WISC-R to somewhat different uses. The neuropsychologist uses the WISC-R to help identify whether there is an organic etiology to the presenting problems of the child. Subtest scores are compared to try to identify the strengths and weaknesses of the child. The school psychologist is more likely to use the WISC-R to predict the highest level of academic achievement possible by an individual child.

The results of the neuropsychological and academic achievement assessment of the child can be combined with reference to the different emphases of the two types of instruments. The neuropsychological evaluation provides information regarding the potential functioning of the child under optimal conditions. As such, these results provide a lower limit to estimates of a child's functioning. The academic achievement testing of the child provides information regarding what the child has been able to learn under the prevailing conditions of the learning situation. By combining the two sets of results, the psychologist can partially determine what factors can promote learning (and more generally, functioning that requires cognitive skill) and what factors impede learning.

Because the neuropsychological evaluation of the child focuses on the level of integrity of discrete cognitive skills, the information provided by such an evaluation may have greater applicability to the design of intervention programs. The psychoeducational evaluation has greater applicability to the diagnosis of specific academic deficiencies. For example, the psychoeducational evaluation may indicate that a child is performing arithmetic skills at a level approximately two standard deviations below the average for the chronological age of the child. The neuropsychological evaluation may then indicate that the deficient performance is secondary to a deficit in understanding spatial relationships among numbers when they are presented in a verbal modality. A remedial educational program can be designed to increase achievement in arithmetic by concentrating on visual displays of the spatial relationships among numbers, coupling that information with verbal representations. Gradually, the visual information is faded in favor of the verbal information. Once the general arithmetic skills have been acquired, the reliance on visual representatiaons would be less necessary. Simultaneously, the school professionals can provide exercises in manipulating spatial relationships in verbal information to increase this skill.

OVERVIEW

It is as easy for a specialist to overlook a problem outside her area of expertise as it is for a generalist to do so. Unfortunately, specialists do not always communicate with each other. It is up to the generalist following the child to make sure that each specialist is aware that the child has been seen by other specialists, and if necessary to act as a conduit for communicating information among the specialists. With this information as background and context, we now turn to an overview of the most commonly seen disorders in children.

2
Developmental Disorders

The terms "developmental disorders" and "developmental delay" usually refer to a wide variety of problems manifested as changes in the orderly progression of the acquisition of skills by the child. There is no single etiology for this group of problems. In fact, for many of the disorders the etiology is unknown. This group includes diagnoses as disparate as mental retardation and hearing disorders. What these problems have in common is that the diagnosis is determined largely by the disjunction between usual development and the stage at which the child presents. In fact it is the presence of a problem in cognitive, sensory, perceptual, or motor functioning in a child in whom the skills cannot be assumed to have been present previously that is the hallmark of developmental disorders, and not the presence of a specific set of symptoms.

There are two main situations under which a developmentally disordered child may present to a general clinician. The first situation occurs when the disorder or delay initially is noticed. The child does not come to the clinician with a diagnosis, but only with a suspicion that something is wrong. For more severe disorders, the initial notice may occur fairly early in life, for example, when the child still does not walk by age two years. For more subtle disorders, the initial notice may not occur until school age, when it becomes apparent that the child is not performing in an age-appropriate fashion in an academic setting.

For some children, the referring question may involve complaints of a behavior disorder or emotional disturbance. The child may act out when he is unable to perform at the same level as his peers. Or as the result of multiple failure experiences, the child may show signs of depressed affect, social withdrawal, and moodiness.

The general child clinician does not possess the specialized skills to diagnose developmental disorders, nor can she reasonably expect to learn to be able to do so without advanced training. However, the general child clinician can learn to be sensitive to the clinical manifestations of these disorders and thereby facilitate referral to a specialist who can perform the diagnosis and initiate appropriate treatment. These children may be misidentified by teachers and parents. The general clinician should learn to listen and observe beyond the presenting complaints to recognize the underlying disorder.

MENTAL RETARDATION

Under DSM-III R, the diagnosis of mental retardation requires a documentation of a subaverage IQ value (lower than 70) as well as evidence of social or vocational impairment. These psychiatric criteria and the legal criteria for obtaining special services for retarded individuals can create a false conception of retardation as a binary, "all-or-none" condition. Nothing could be further from the truth. Many different levels of intellectual functioning are possible, and only slightly fewer possible values of IQ. The American Association on Mental Deficiency (AAMD) also more generally defines mental retardation as significant subaverage intellectual functioning with deficits in adaptive functioning manifested during the developmental period. The inclusion of criteria regarding deficits in adaptive functioning allows some flexibility in assigning a diagnosis of mental retardation.

A collection of behavioral symptoms are associated with diagnoses of mental retardation. These children may exhibit behavioral passivity and dependence. They may also engage in stereotyped self-stimulatory or self-injurious behavior. In addition, mentally retarded children may exhibit a low tolerance for change or for frustration. They can have a poor self image. Frequently they will show impulsiveness both in the free environment and during testing procedures. For all of these reasons, mentally retarded children are at risk for behavioral and emotional disturbances and may need psychological intervention.

Children with very low IQs are likely to be diagnosed early in life. Children with more subtle forms of retardation may remain undetected for years, during which the child experiences failure, social censure from peers, frustration over lack of progress, and punishment from unwittingly misunderstanding parents and teachers. Therefore, one of the most important parts of any evaluation of a child includes an IQ test, preferably one that is recognized by the legal system so as to help the child obtain services. Quick estimates of IQ are not helpful in these cases except to indicate the need for a standard IQ test. We recommend that the clinician use the WISC-R, Stanford-Binet, or some other comprehensive intelligence test at the beginning.

Sometimes the clinician is faced with a difficult ethical question in diagnosing children who just meet the IQ requirements but whose social functioning is borderline. The ethical questions are raised because of the consequences of labelling. Some diagnoses, such as childhood measles, have minimal consequences for the self-esteem of the child and are easily forgotten over time. Other diagnoses, such as mental retardation, carry many meanings for both the child and parents and these tend to persist and even become permanent qualifiers on what is expected of an individual.

The clinician is well advised to consider carefully the consequences of diagnosis and to discuss these consequences with the parents. This is not to say that the clinician should allow the desires of the parents to determine clinical practice. However, if a child is performing reasonably well in school, appears not to be in need of special services, and has adequate interpersonal adjustment, the diagnosis of mental retardation should be given second and third thoughts. Although it is unlikely that such a child would be referred for evaluation in the first place, it is possible and does happen.

The astute reader has noticed that the diagnosis of mental retardation leaves the etiology unspecified. This omission arises fom the fact that the etiologies of mental retardation are varied. Mental retardation can result from causes as diverse as nutritional insufficiency, genetic transmission, prenatal or perinatal factors, infectious disease in early childhood, or trauma to the brain. There are those clinicians who do not consider childhood brain trauma to be a cause of mental retardation, but rather a separate entity. However, due to the diagnostic definition of mental retardation, the two are not mutually exclusive. This is a very different situation from that in adults.

When adults experience lowered IQ as the result of a brain trauma, the diagnosis given them is usually "dementia." Although this designation is no more useful in understanding the individual than the diagnosis of "mental retardation" in the child, the use of the term dementia does point out the requirement that the cognitive impairment is acquired following a premorbid period in which the individual demonstrated evidence of higher levels of cognitive skills. For the child who experiences early brain trauma, such evidence may be lacking. For a young child, there is little opportunity to show vocational or social adaptation. The exceptions are in school-age children who suffered trama after they had already completed a few years of school.

The solution may be in a nosological, diagnostic system that has greater specificity in etiological diagnosis and in description of current level of various skills. In the meanwhile, it is useful to remember that the diagnosis of mental retardation may not provide the clinician with information regarding the best treatment of the child or with useful predictions regarding the child's behavior. For example, a child with Down syndrome and a child with a head injury may both have the same IQ. However, the child with Down syndrome may exhibit the characteristic gentle and compliant behavior whereas the child with the head injury may show impulsive and possibly aggressive behavior.

Rather than relying on the diagnosis of the child, the clinician should be cognizant of the etiology. When in doubt, the clinician can consult a specialist. A pediatric neurologist or a pediatrician may provide useful information regarding the medical complications of a given etiological diagnosis while a child neuropsychologist may provide useful information regarding the cognitive and interpersonal development of the child with that etiological diagnosis.

Earlier, a small sample of etiologies possibly responsible for mental retardation was given. However, the range of etiologies is even larger than that. A wide variety of morphological, physiological, metabolic, and chemical problems can result in mental retardation if they occur in the prenatal, perinatal, or even postnatal periods. Prenatal etiologic agents include maternal rubella (German measles), toxoplasmosis, and syphilis. Etiological agents with effects in early life include birth trauma (especially if it results in anoxic episodes) and metabolic conditions such as hyperbilirubinemia and hypoglycemia.

In early life, cerebral functions are sensitive to environmental events and agents to a degree that is not matched until much later in life. Both very young and very old individuals are most susceptible to the cerebral effects of infections, trauma, intoxication, exposure to neurotoxins, and postimmunization encephalopathies. Finally and most sadly, mental retardation can be the result of psychosocial factors when these result in deprivation of the infant or child.

GENETIC DISORDERS

There are a number of genetic disorders that can result in cognitive impairment. Some of the more common are phenylketonuria, Turner's Syndrome, and Down Syndrome.

Phenylketonuria

The genetics of phenylketonuria (PKU) are presented in high-school biology classes. PKU is perhaps the most common of the genetic disorders that result in mental retardation. In children with PKU, an enzyme that usually metabolizes phenylalanine is absent due to a genetic abnormality. Phenylalanine builds up in the tissues of the child and slows the development of nervous tissue. The cognitive features of PKU include mental retardation, a limited attention span, and a lower level of responsiveness to environmental events than is found in unafflicted children. During the medical evaluation, these children present a history of seizures and show the symptoms of spasticity, abnormally high reflexes, tremor, and abnormal EEGs. The children tend to be short in stature; have light colored hair, eyes, and skin; have smaller than average hands; and may develop dermatitis. Their behavior tends to be restless and hyperactive. Their parents describe them as hyperactive, destructive, and irritable.

Treatment of PKU is a restricted diet that minimizes the buildup of phenylalanine. This diet involves limiting the intake of proteins and may cause some problems related to protein deficiency. It is unclear just how long the diet needs to be maintained. Some studies have been interpreted as evidence for the need for long-term diets, whereas other data have been invoked to support the existence of iatrogenic protein deficiency secondary to the restricted diet. One point is clear, however; the management of a child with PKU requires the cooperation of child psychologists and pediatric specialists. Psychologists are needed to follow the development of the child, to document changes in intellectual functioning, and to provide consultation to the parents regarding behavioral management. Medical specialists are needed to assess regularly blood levels of phenylalanine and to suggest changes in the diet.

Turner's Syndrome

Turner's syndrome is the result of a deficiency in sex-linked chromosomes. Specifically, the child with Turner's syndrome is missing one chromosome and has only one sex chromosome, the X chromosome. In appearance, the child with Turner's syndrome is a female with short stature. However, the primary sex characteristics are poorly developed, and the individuals are sterile. Generally, these children are not mentally retarded, although their IQs may be slightly lower than average. Children with Turner's syndrome show characteristic deficits in spatial relationships which appear to be related more to visual perceptual than to constructional abilities. These children also show deficits in attention. There has been much speculation as to the etiology of this spatial deficit in Turner's syndrome children, ranging from structural deficits in the right parietal region to lack of sex-linked lateralization for speech functions. Recent empirical evidence suggests that focal central nervous system dysfunction cannot explain the pattern of deficits found in these children (McGlone, 1985).

The exact etiology of these deficits is relatively unimportant in the care that a general clinician can provide for a child with Turner's syndrome. Because most of these children demonstrate average IQ levels, their academic problems in school related to their spatial deficits may be overlooked or misattributed to motivational factors. By referring for a complete neuropsychological evaluation, the clinician can help obtain information regarding the best approach to educating the child. It is also important to remember that due to the sex chromosomal abnormalities, many of these children will show adjustment problems during puberty. The clinician can provide the family with factual information and with a model of understanding toward the child and her special problems.

Down Syndrome

The Down syndrome (also known as Mongolism or trisomy 21) include mental retardation and other physical abnormalities such as anomalous skeletal growth. These children have a flattened face with a small and rounded skull, their eyes are slanted with epicanthal folds, and their tongues are elongated and protruding. They are usually of normal size at birth but soon fall behind the growth curve. There is an associated congenital cardiac malformation that becomes fatal in early adulthood.

The cause of Down syndrome is usually a triplication of chromosome 21. Another cause is translocation of chromosome 21. Although this is a genetic disorder, it is not always inherited. It tends to be more common in children born to older mothers, although it can occur in children born to mothers of any age. The diagnosis is usually made at birth. Children with Down syndrome have a gentle demeanor and are quite docile and responsive to affection. Intellectual functioning, although generally impaired, can range from minor impairment to severe retardation.

The role of the general child clinician is to assess the intellectual functioning of the child and help plan education and psychological interventions. Parents may be overprotective of these children, and the clinician should encourage the parents to challenge their children to perform independently as many functions as possible. Treatment of the child is symptomatic. Counseling the parents is more involved. It includes supportive therapy as well as consultation in managing the child. Because this is a congenital condition, parents often react to the disorder with feelings of guilt or embarrassment. There may also be elements of denial, especially when the child is still very young. The parents may need initial help in accepting the diagnosis and continued help in dealing with coming to grips with many features of the disorder, especially the early death of most of the children.

EXPOSURE TO NEUROTOXINS

Exposure to neurotoxins, both prenatally and postnatally, is probably underestimated as a problem to our society. It is likely that due to the long-term effects of chronic exposure, many neurotoxins are as yet unidentified. Even with the identified neurotoxins, such as lead, there may be a highly dangerous level of exposure. Recently, the problem of lead exposure has been addressed by governmental agencies. It is unfortunate that many of the children exposed to lead in the form of old wall paint are more likely to engage in pica because of nutritional deficits in their own diets. However, it is not only the inner-city child who eats lead paint from the peeling walls of his apartment who is at risk. It is also the middle-class child whose family lives in close proximity to foundries or battery factories. Children exposed to lead may show mental retardation, decreased reflexes, weakness, and slow nerve conduction studies, probably secondary to demyelination (removal of insulating lipid structures from around the sheath of the axon).

Still another unfortunate situation of exposure to neurotoxins results from the use of insecticides or herbicides. This is more common in rural or suburban children but is not unknown in urban children. The exposure may result from unwitting parental use of insecticides in the back yard. Children play at ground level and may show the effects of exposure even when adults in the same household do not. Older children who roam when they play may be exposed to insecticides in a favorite field. Insecticides are designed to have staying power and the field need not have been recently sprayed to have an effect. Parents should be advised to monitor carefully their children's play environments to prevent problems.

VITAMIN AND OTHER NUTRITIONAL DEFICIENCIES

Sadly, nutritional deficiencies are not limited to children in developing nations. Nutritional deficiencies can occur wherever the diet of children is neglected—in the children of two working parents who do not take the time to provide an adequate diet, or in the children of parents who do not feel that the fight over diet is worth the effort. An old study frequently cited by nutritional laissez-faire proponents concluded that children left to their own devices will spontaneously pick an adequately balanced diet. That study was conducted before the age of fast foods and empty calorie snack foods. In addition, the free diet from which the children in the study were allowed to choose contained a large proportion of healthy foods such as fresh fruits and vegetables. Any assumption that a child will spontaneously balance his own diet is probably untenable.

Thiamine (vitamin B_1) is a precursor of one of the coenzymes in carbohydrate metabolism, and may be implicated in peripheral nerve conduction. Thiamine has a quick turnover in the body and therefore is not stored for long. Dietary restriction of thiamine can result in a deficiency sufficient to cause clinical symptoms in less than three months. Many conditions other than dietary restriction can reduce the levels of thiamine in the body. These include diarrhea and colitis in the infant, liver dysfunction, intestinal parasites, fever, infection, and diuresis. Teenage girls on strict self-imposed diets are at risk for developing thiamine deficiencies. Another factor to be considered in teenagers is the role of alcohol in reducing body levels of thiamine.

The early signs of thiamine deficiency include irritability, anorexia, and weight loss. These individuals may complain of sensitivity to noise, decreased concentration, anxiety, depression, insomnia, or parathesias. Later there may be signs of ataxia, edema, or peripheral neuropathy. The mamillary bodies are not usually affected by thiamine deficiencies in children, and this may be one reason why loss of memory secondary to thiamine deficiency is not as common in children as in adults.

Thiamine is found in cereals, legumes, nuts, potatoes, eggs, and meat. A clinician who suspects thiamine deficiency can inquire as to recent infections, fevers, or changes in diet. Thiamine deficiencies can be reversible with medical treatment, so quick referral to a medical specialist may help avoid later, irreversible problems with mental deficiency.

Clinically, two frequently discussed nutritional deficiencies are *kwashiorkor* (protein deficiency) and *marasmus* (calorie deficiency). The reader can consult the chapter on the interview and history for a more complete discussion of these two disorders. Both of these can occur in children consuming a diet that is otherwise sufficient. Other dietary insufficiencies include vitamin A deficiency, which is a cause of blindness. These disorders are quite dramatic when seen in their complete clinical manifestations. However, it is important to remember that these disorders do not suddenly occur when the level of specific substances in the diet of a child dips below a certain level. Children, especially the very young, are more sensitive to deficiencies in their diets than are adults (with the exception of the elderly who again show this sensitivity). It is important for the clinician faced with a case of cognitive difficulty or developmental delay to inquire as to the diet of the child. When there are any doubts, the child should be sent for a medical evaluation with the suspicions communicated to the physician. Most nutritional deficiency based developmental delays can be reversed with timely changes in diet or with the use of nutritional supplements. The general clinician may be the first professional to see a child with this problem, and quick action may be necessary.

Maternal use of alcohol has been briefly discussed in the context of the chapter on taking a history. A few more comments are in order. Previously it was thought that heavy use of alcohol by a pregnant woman was necessary to cause the low birth weight, frequency of failure to thrive, presence of neurological soft signs, and later learning disabilities associated with the fetal alcohol syndrome. However, it is important to remember that rather than a minimum level of alcohol use needed to produce the effects, there is probably a dose-dependent relationship between the amount of alcohol used by a pregnant woman and the effects sometimes seen. Another consideration is the relationship between maternal smoking and birth weight. It is best for a pregnant woman to avoid alcohol and cigarette smoking altogether.

SENSORY DISORDERS

Some children may exhibit deficits in basic sensory functions as they relate to audition, visual processes, or tactile sensation. Sensory deficits may be due to lesions anywhere in the sensory system, including the receptor organ, the peripheral nerve route, or the central nervous system. Before assuming a central nervous system etiology for a sensory dysfunction, it is necessary to rule out dysfunction earlier in the chain. In addition, different areas of the brain appear to be responsible for adequate processing of sensory information. For example, visual problems may be due to lesions in the lateral geniculate nucleus which acts as a relay station for visual information. Visual problems may also be due to lesions in regions of the occipital lobe responsible for visual perception.

Peripheral receptor organ difficulties that have a central nervous system etiology include disorders of lateral conjugate gaze. Here paired movements of the eyes upward and downward and from side to side are disturbed, as are eye movements involved in convergence and divergence so important to the perception of spatial location of an object. *Nystagmus* or short involuntary, rhythmic movements of the eyes may also cause difficulties in accurate visual sensation. *Strabismus,* the condition of being cross-eyed, can similarly impact in visual sensation.

Lesions in the occipital lobes may cause visual field defects. Here some portion of the visual field is not perceived. The area of imperception is called a *scotoma.* If the occipital lesions are responsible, the deficits will be the same for each eye. A field cut encompassing one quarter of the visual field is called a *quandrantonopia.* A field cut encompassing one-half of the visual field is called a *hemianopia.* Large lesions of the occipital lobes may cause cortical blindness. It is common that an individual overlooks or attempts to compensate for his visual defects. An extreme example of this is known as Anton's syndrome, where the cortically blind patient denies any visual problems and confabulates to try and cover for the deficit. This form of denial is more common in patients with visual deficits than in patients with other sensory deficits. Although the concept may at first seem bizarre, it becomes more understandable when we consider our own covering for, and inattention, the ubiquitous blind spot.

There are other, more complicated forms of visual impairment more related to perceptual processes than to direct sensory processes. Visual agnosia occurs when an individual can sense but not recognize visual material. Visual discrimination is intact, but visual recognition is impaired. Color perception or recognition may also be impaired. Lesions in higher order perceptual centers may cause deficits in visual spatial relationships. Blind children are in need of extra stimulation to obviate common delays in motor, sensory, and social development.

AUDITORY DISORDERS

Auditory processing appears to be separately represented for verbal and nonverbal material. Children with auditory deficits may show delays in language acquisition as well as in social development. Auditory disorders are frequently accompanied by motor difficulties or cognitive impairment. Emotional disorders are seen with only moderate levels of frequency in these children. Children with higher order auditory perceptual disorders may not be diagnosed until the developmental age at which these skills are called into use. For example, deficits in auditory recognition but not auditory discrimination will not be noticed until the child shows difficulty in acquiring language skills.

LANGUAGE DISORDERS

Language acquisition is an important aspect of normal development. Our culture is heavily verbal, and children with language delays are at significant risk for problems in other areas. As seen above, sensory deficits can delay language acquisition. Language disorders shown by children include total deficits, delayed development, and loss of previously acquired skills. Most children show some form of language acquisition by the age of four years and failure to do so is a cause for concern. Language delays are often seen in connection with other developmental disorders such as mental retardation. Developmental language delays appear to have a genetic component as they tend to run in families.

Language disorders may be specific to either receptive or expressive speech. The receptive deficits may be specific to the recognition of morphemes, the understanding of words, or to the comprehension of meaning from syntactical or grammatical information. Expressive speech deficits may be related to pronunciation (articulation), to appropriate word usage (semantic paraphasia), to the ability to produce grammatically correct sequences, or to the ability to group words into meaningful units. Language disordered children may have associated intellectual deficits, although this is not a universal phenomenon.

The DSM-III R contains categories for the diagnosis of language disorders when those disorders are the result of developmental delays. These categories are under the general heading of specific developmental disorders and include Developmental Expressive Writing Disorder, Developmental Reading Disorder, Developmental Articulation Disorder, and Developmental Expressive Language Disorder. In each of these cases the etiology cannot be related to peripheral sensory disorders, mental retardation, or a neurological disorder. It is important to remember that the symptoms of, for example, an expressive language disorder may occur in a child with a history of head injury; the DSM-III R diagnosis of Developmental Expressive Language Disorder cannot be assigned in this case. Similarly, there may be differences in the optimal treatment of disorders arising from the two different etiologies. If the clinician will be following the child for treatment purposes, consultation with a child neuropsychologist is necessary to choose the most appropriate treatment.

OVERVIEW

The general child clinician will not regularly see the full panoply of developmental disorders. However, there are two situations in which a general child clinician may see children with developmental disorders. In the first case a child with a diagnosed developmental disorder is brought to the clinician because of problems in academic achievement or behavioral-emotional adjustment. Here the clinician should be cognizant of the usual presentation of the particular disorder to help design an intervention system consistent with the deficits of the child. The second situation involves those children for whom a diagnosis has not yet been given, but for whom some problems have been identified. Here the clinician should be sensitive to the possibility of a developmental disorder to help facilitate referral to an appropriate specialist. In neither case can the general child clinician remain ignorant of the different disorders possible.

3
Neurological Disorders of Childhood

Children with neurological disorders are referred to child clinicians for several different reasons. In some instances, the underlying neurological disorder may not be diagnosed at the time of referral. The child clinician must be alert to the possibility of a neurological disorder on the basis of the obtained history or clinical presentation and then refer to an appropriate specialist. In other instances, the neurological disorder may have been diagnosed, but the psychological concomitants may not be understood by the parents or teachers. Here the role of the clinician is to educate the parents and teachers as to how the disorder is affecting the behavior and cognitive development of the child. In some of these cases, it may also be necessary to link up the medical specialists with the neuropsychological specialist to provide optimum care for the child. In yet another set of circumstances, the diagnosis and possible psychological concomitants are known, but the parents desire documentation of the exact level of cognitive and psychological deficit to help plan educational and other interventions.

In any of these cases, the clinician should be aware of some of the more common psychological aspects of neurological disorders to be better able to plan an assessment, recognize a disorder, or plan an intervention. This chapter should be viewed as only a starting point in the understanding of these principles. The general clinician should consult a reference library or a specialist possessing the requisite information.

SEIZURE DISORDERS

In children, as in adults, the seizure disorders are better conceptualized as symptoms rather than as diseases. A wide variety of neurological problems can cause seizure disorders. Many of these problems are shared with adults. However, the relative prevalence of different etiologies changes with age. For example, the most common causes of recent onset of a seizure disorder in an adult is a tumor, cerebral-vascular accident, or trauma. In infants, the most common causes include toxemia or infection, congenital defects, or metabolic deficiency. In children the most prevalent causes are fever, infectious disease, or trauma. In elderly adults, the most common cause is some form of metabolic disorder. Idiopathic seizure disorders, that is, seizures unrelated to some environmental or other diagnosable entity, appear for the first time more commonly in children than in adults. There may be genetic causes of these idiopathic seizure disorders.

The exact relationship between seizure disorders and the level of neuropsychological skill of an individual is still being investigated. However, it is probably safe to say that the level of neuropsychological skill is inversely correlated to the lifelong number of seizure episodes. Children with uncontrollable seizure disorders may exhibit declines in intellectual functioning over time. The presence of these deficits needs to be documented by baseline psychological and follow-up evaluations. A single episode of febrile seizure or afrebile convulsions is not strictly a seizure disorder, but it should be noted that although the appearance of either of these two in an infant may have no significant impact on later cognitive abilities, multiple occurrences of such episodes may be responsible for later cognitive deficits.

This is not to say that epileptic children will not be in the bright range of intellectual functioning. It is possible that a child with epilepsy may show no signs of impairment on intellectual assessment. On the other hand, it may be that a more focused neuropsychological evaluation may uncover subtle deficits of either a specific or diffuse nature. Not enough is known about epilepsy for us to make (or accept) any broad statements about the neuropsychological functioning of an epileptic child. Therefore, the evaluation of an epileptic child should not be biased by any preconceptions held by the clinician.

There are several different classification systems for the diagnoses of seizure disorders. Table 3-1 lists some of the seizure disorders that are possible in children. The classification system in Table 3-1 is a modification of the system suggested by the Internation League Against Epilepsy (ILAE, 1981) and a system suggested by Tharp (1987).

The types of seizure disorders exhibited by children include localization-related epilepsy. These are sometimes known by the names *focal, local,* or *partial* epilepsy. Here the seizure is secondary to some documented or presumed lesion limited to a certain area of the brain. The psychological and motor consequences of these seizures are usually characteristically related to the area of the brain exhibiting the spike abnormalities. For example, childhood temporal lobe epilepsy may be associated with some of

TABLE 3-1 Classification System for Childhood Seizure Disorders

I. Localization related seizures (focal, local, partial)
   A. Idiopathic with age-related onset
   B. Symptomatic
      1. Simple partial seizures (with motor, somatosensory, autonomic, or psychological symptoms)
      2. Simple partial (with impairment of consciousness)
      3. Partial seizures evolving to generalized

II. Generalized seizures (convulsive or nonconvulsive)
   A. Idiopathic with age-related onset
   B. Absence seizures (with impairment of consciousness, mild clonic, atonic, or tonic components, automatisms, or autonomic components)
   C. Atypical absence
   D. Myoclonic seizures (single or multiple jerks)
   E. Tonic seizures
   F. Clonic seizures
   G. Tonic-clonic (grand mal)
   H. Atonic seizures

III. Unclassified seizure disorders

---

the same symptoms associated with the adult form, namely, garrulousness, irritability, and overconcern with religious matters. The symptomatology of simple-partial seizures may include motor signs, sensory or somatosensory signs, or autonomic nervous system signs. Complex-partial syndromes may have associated disturbances of consciousness, automatisms, or cognitive, affective, or psychosensory symptoms.

One form of seizure disorder that is frequently undetected or misunderstood by parents and teachers is the *absence* seizure. Here the major symptom may be a temporary aberration in normal consciousness. The child's face may become blank (the "blank stare") for a short period of time during which the child is largely unresponsive to external stimulation. The child may be embarrassed or frightened by the episodes and may not fully explain the experience to adults. Frequently, adults interpret the behavior as willful inattention or daydreaming. The presenting complaint may be daydreaming or poor academic achievement. When an absence seizure is suspected, the child clinician should refer the child to a pediatric neurologist for a more complete evaluation.

Generalized seizures include *petit mal* (the absence seizures discussed above), *myoclonic* (or "muscle jerk"), *infantile spasms, akinetic* seizures, and the motor seizures of *tonic, clonic, and tonic-clonic* (grand mal) seizures with their major motor symptoms. Idiopathic seizures are not well understood, but there may be some genetic factor involved, as a family history positive for seizure disorders is associated with the occurrence of the disorder.

The reasons for referral to a child clinician usually center around emotional-behavioral adjustment or educational planning. There might be multiple reasons for the behavioral problems sometimes reported in epileptic children. Some theorists speculate that the abnormal brain electrical activity responsible for the epilepsy may also be responsible for behavioral abnormalities. Other theorists state that the different treatment of the epileptic child coupled with the identification of the child as different by peers and adults may be responsible for the psychological difficulties (Bolter, 1986). Whatever the cause, it is generally accepted that epileptic children exhibit a more frequent manifestation of psychopathology than do nonepileptic children. These children are more likely to be referred to a child clinician than is the average child.

Despite the fact that epilepsy appears to be a strictly medical disorder, there are many psychological factors that are important to consider in the treatment of these children. Seizures can be brought on by a lack of sleep, changes in level of environmental stress, or any of a number of environmental variables. Sometimes a child will become conditioned to certain contextual variables in eliciting seizure behavior. These contextual variables may include setting (school vs. home) and the presence of certain individuals, such as the mother, during the seizure episode. The response of significant others to the seizures can increase or decrease their frequency. In addition, the extra effort and care that accompanies management of a seizure disorder can have an effect on the adjustment of the child and on the relationships among family members. The general child clinician, by working closely with a pediatric neurologist, can help augment the medical treatment of the child with psychological care.

HYDROCEPHALUS

Hydrocephalus is a condition in which there is a buildup of fluids in the brain of the child. There are two general forms of hydrocephalus: noncommunicating (or obstructive) and communicating (normal pressure or occult). In noncommunicating hydrocephalus, some form of obstruction of the normal flow of cerebrospinal fluid (CSF) occurs. This can be due to a lesion in the ventricular system, to a stenosis (narrowing) of the Sylvian aqueduct, or to cysts and tumors.

In normal pressure hydrocephalus, there is some dysfunction of the absorbing functions of the arachnoid villae, the structures responsible for removing CSF from the ventricular system. More rarely, normal pressure hydrocephalus may be due to oversecretion of CSF caused by a choroid plexus papilloma. The internal pressure of the ventricle system remains constant (hence the name). To maintain the pressure and still accommodate the increases in fluid quantity, the brain becomes compressed with a resultant decrease in the efficiency with which brain functions are conducted. It should be pointed out that many cases of chronic hydrocephalus are not associated with eithier motor or cognitive impairment (Caviness, 1987).

Normal pressure hydrocephalus develops over time. The features become apparent gradually. Clinical features of normal pressure hydrocephalus include decline in intellectual function. Children may show regressions in developmental stage. They may become listless or appear to be depressed. Memory functions start to fail. In an adult, normal pressure hydrocephalus is accompanied by a triad of ataxia, incontinence, and dementia. Although these signs may also be present in children, normal pressure hydrocephalus is usually detected on the basis of failure to meet developmental milestones, motor clumsiness, or increases in head size beyond the normal growth curve.

Normal pressure hydrocephalus in children is usually treated by surgical implant of a shunt that diverts the CSF to another cavity in the body, usually the abdominal cavity where it is then absorbed by the body. Following the placement of a successful shunt, the clinical signs are usually reversed. Currently, pre- and postsurgical evaluation of normal pressure hydrocephalus generally includes an intellectual evaluation. However, a more complete neuropsychological evaluation is recommended because many of the motor and specific cognitive deficits may not be identified by an intellectual evaluation.

TOURETTE SYNDROME

Tourette syndrome is a disorder that sits at the juncture among neurology, psychiatry, and psychology. There is an interaction among the neurophysiological, genetic, behavioral, and environmental factors that changes the manifestation of the disorder across the developmental cycle. Because of the idiosyncratic behavioral manifestations of Tourette syndrome, there is much interest in the disorder. Unfortunately, there is also much misunderstanding.

Specifically, Tourette syndrome is a lifelong disorder that waxes and wanes with time and that may be sensitive to environmental factors such as the level of experienced stress. The outstanding characteristic of Tourette syndrome is the tic, which tends to be a combination of behaviors that may involve simple tics of small muscle groups (grimaces or nose twitching), small stereotyped behavioral chains (such as picking at one's clothing), or outbursts of scatalogical language. In some instances the tic involves animal sounds such as barking. It can be a cause of significant embarrassment to the individual.

The child with Tourette syndrome, usually a boy, exhibits normal intelligence. However, this child often shows deficits in visual-motor integration tasks. The child tends to have problems in academic performance which are probably secondary to deficits in sustained attention and to psychological adjustment difficulties rather than directly secondary to the tics. Hyperactivity and impulse control difficulties also have been reported in conjunction with Tourette syndrome.

As well as the psychological adjustment problems mentioned earlier, the Tourette syndrome child often shows features of obsessive-compulsive behaviors. Frequently, the symptoms of obsessive-compulsive behavior, hyperactivity, and impulse control deficits appear prior to the first tic activity. A general clinician may therefore be the first health care professional to come into contact with a child with Tourette syndrome. When in doubt, referral to a specialist is in order.

The diagnosis of Tourette syndrome requires a complete physical examination and neurological evaluation as well as laboratory testing such as an EEG. The laboratory testing is necessary to rule out other possible diagnoses, as Tourette syndrome does not show a characteristic pattern of test results. The treatment of Tourette syndrome usually involves administration of haloperidol although pimozide or clonidine is also used. Medical management is typically provided by a pediatric neurologist or child psychiatrist. The general clinician who suspects Tourette syndrome can help provide information regarding the diagnosis by assessing the situations and time periods associated with the tic activity. Because there has been a high degree of associated family and psychological adjustment problems, the general child clinician can help provide some of the needed intervention in these cases.

Tics are quick, rhythmic, involuntary, and purposeless movements of single muscle groups. Tic disorders are sometimes confused with Tourette syndrome, and in fact the relationship between the two may be more a matter of both existing along a continuum (Williams, Pleak, & Hanesian, 1987). Tic disorders can also be embarrassing to the afflicted individual. In general, a child with a tic disorder, particularly a transient tic disorder, exhibits fewer adjustment and academic problems than a child with Tourette syndrome. It is wise to evaluate for the presence of these problems.

MUSCULAR DYSTROPHIES

Muscular dystrophies are a mixed group of disorders that share features of being degenerative, involving weakness of skeletal muscles and exhibition of bilateral atrophy. There are many different types of muscular dystrophy, and the etiology of most is unknown. The three most common forms in children are *Duchenne muscular dystrophy* (an X chromosome-linked autosomal recessive disorder), *Becker type* (an X-linked disorder that has a later onset and slower progression than Duchenne), *Landouzy–Dejerine type* (an autosomal dominant disorder), *Steinert dystrophy* (an autosomal dominant disorder with onset from childhood to adulthood), and *congenital muscular dystrophy* (possibly autosomal recessive). Differing degrees of mental retardation have been reported in Duchenne, Steinert, and congenital muscular dystrophies. There have been less frequent reports of mental retardation associated with the other muscular dystrophies.

The most common form of muscular dystrophy is Duchenne, which occurs more frequently in males. The first symptoms of Duchenne appear between the ages of two and four years, when delays in developmental milestones become apparent. The child shows difficulty in running and walking and may fall frequently. The gait appears to be a form of waddling. Later the child shows difficulty in lifting his arms above his head. By the time the child reaches the teen years, he is usually required to use a wheelchair for ambulation. Death from respiratory failure or pneumonia typically occurs before the age of 30.

Becker type is also more common in males, but it has a later onset than does Duchenne, and the progression is slower. These individuals may live to be 50 years old before dying of the complications. Also cardiac abnormalities are not as common here as in Duchenne. Landouzy–Dejerine type is even more slowly progressive, with the first features occurring between 6 and 20 years of age. In Landouzy–Dejerine there may also be periods of time during which the progression is halted.

OTHER DISORDERS OF NEUROMUSCULAR DEVELOPMENT

Motor disorders can occur from a wide variety of etiologies including prenatal toxemia, infection, or hemorrhage. Premature and low-birth-weight infants, very young children with perinatal trauma or hemorrhage, infants who experience hypoxia, and children who experience perinatal seizures are all at risk to develop disorders of neuromuscular development. Symptoms can include paralysis and muscle weakness, *spasticity* (resistance to movement coupled with abnormal reflexes and hypertonia), dystonia and athetosis (abnormal involuntary twisting of limbs and trunk), choreiform movements, rigidity (increased muscle tone), ataxia (difficulty in maintaining balance and in performing fine motor activity), and tremor.

The major symptoms of disorders of neuromuscular development are motor deficits but will often include associated deficits in tactile sensation, lowered intelligence, and delays in speech development. These associated symptoms do not always occur, but they do occur with enough frequency to warrant screening these children for the presence of neuropsychological deficits.

CEREBRAL PALSY

Cerebral palsy is a somewhat nonspecific diagnosis used for people who exhibit muscle weakness, spasticity, or other inaccuracies of the control of motor activity, and ataxia. There are many different causes of cerebral palsy, but all of them occur either during the birth process or shortly thereafter. Some individuals with cerebral palsy may exhibit a degree of mental retardation, but this is not true of all cases. Because of the variability in etiology and presentation of cerebral palsy, a complete neuropsychological evaluation is necessary before psychological treatment or academic intervention is initiated.

HEAD INJURY

Perhaps one of the most common causes of neurological dysfunction in children is head injury. Head trauma may account for as much as 43% of all deaths in children aged five to nine years. Unlike the situation in adults, the majority of cases in children are due to causes other than motor vehicle accidents. Falling accidents account for between 55 and 65% of head injuries in children (Rivara & Mueller, 1986). Child abuse accounts for an unsubstantiated but probably significant percentage of child head injuries. In older children and adolescents, sports-related accidents cause many head injuries.

There are several mechanisms by which head injury can result in damage to the brain. Contusion can be thought of as a bruise on the brain. Small blood vessels become torn and blood leaks out into the brain. If the contusion is well-circumscribed, the child may show focal signs, although as noted above brain damage in children results more frequently in diffuse signs. Lacerations are large rips or tears in brain tissue and are more likely to result from penetrating wounds than from closed head injury. The neuropsychological effects of lacerations are more severe than those of contusions. If in a closed head injury large blood vessels have been torn, pools of blood may accumulate in areas of the brain, especially in the meninges. This is known as hematoma. Subdural hematoma can be especially dangerous because the effects are not always noticeable immediately following the injury. Later the child may complain of nausea and over the course of several hours may develop neurological symptoms or loss of consciousness. If untreated, hematoma can result in death. Although hematoma are unlikely to be seen by general child clinicians in their acute form, any suggestion of hematoma is reason for immediate referral for emergency treatment.

Shear strain injury results from acceleration/deceleration accidents. Here the brain is moving at a given speed and suddenly decelerates hitting a solid surface such as the dashboard of an automobile. The axons are stretched and depolarized even if they are not actually torn. This results in inefficient electrochemical activity and diffuse cognitive deficits. Shear strain injuries are more likely to affect neurotransmission through layers of the same brain area, although the neural connections across brain areas may also be affected.

The traditional wisdom has held that head injury results in less severe behavioral sequelae in children than in adults. However, like much of clinical lore, empirical evidence is wanting on this point. The skull of a young child is less rigid than that of an adult, and therefore may absorb more of the physical injury. However, the lesser rigidity also may result in greater distortion of the brain during an injury and, therefore, greater shear (sliding of brain tissue over other tissue) strain damage (Rutter, Chadwick, & Shaffer 1983).

It is important to remember that many different factors impinge upon the sequelae of brain injury including age at occurrence, type of injury including the physics of the injury, developmental age at injury, and sex of the child. The best course is to evaluate skills across a wide range of functions following a head injury rather than assume the nature of its effects. It should also be remembered that the effects of brain injury are more generalized in children than in adults. Sometimes, the results of an early head injury may not be totally noticeable for a few years after the injury. This is particularly true if the injuries damage an area of the brain that was not totally developed. For example, early injury to the frontal lobes may not exhibit the full range of deficits until later in life when the child's cohorts start exhibiting age-appropriate abstraction skills and the frontal-lobe-injured child does not.

Although there is currently a debate regarding the effects of minor head injury, it is possible that earlier conclusions regarding the lack of neuropsychological effects may have been due to the use of insufficiently sensitive assessment techniques. Effects of minor head injury may include attention difficulties, deficits in the transfer of information from short-term to long-term memory, and personality change. If a head injury is suspected, the clinician should attempt to gather as much information as possible, including whether and for how long a period there was a loss of consciousness, whether any changes in academic performance are temporally related to the injury, the extent of medical care required for treatment of the injury, and whether seizure episodes followed the injury.

For the first six months following head injury the child may show generalized and pervasive deficits, the most prominent of which is memory complaints. Another common effect of head injury in children is visual spatial impairment. Head injuries in adults as well as in children can interfere with the acquisition of new information. This can be unfortunate in adults, but it is even more disastrous in children who have not yet acquired much of the information they will need for optimal adjustment. In a sense, the child's learning is discontinued, fixating him at a certain level.

Children who experience head injury are at greater risk for intellectual impairment, behavioral disorders, and emotional adjustment difficulties. These children often require special educational services. Sometimes parents and teachers may not be aware of the neuropsychological sequelae of a head injury. At other times the child may not have told the parents about a playground injury. The general child clinician should be aware of the possible effects of head injury and should inquire as to the presence of a head injury in the history of the child and screen for memory, visual spatial, and intellectual problems in these children. Recent changes in academic functioning, behavioral patterns, or emotional adjustment should be reason enough to investigate the possibility that a head injury has occurred.

OVERVIEW

There are many different forms of neurological disorders, both diagnosed and undiagnosed, that can result in referral to a general child clinician. Although the clinician cannot possibly be expert in detecting all of these disorders or in assessing the effects of the disorders, some familiarity with the type of disorders and types of neuropsychological effects can improve the level of care provided to the child.

Many childhood head injuries are potentially preventable. This fact is both a cause of regret and a reason for hope. By educating parents, the child clinician can help reduce the incidence of head injury in children. Many states now require some form of safety restraint for children traveling in automobiles. Parents should be encouraged to use these restraints. Increased levels of supervision for young children just beginning to cruise can reduce the frequently of accidents. The use of hall gates set at stairways can also reduce child head injuries. Playground activity and sports, especially football, should be supervised. Finally, if the clinician suspects child abuse or neglect, quick action can facilitate interventions with the parents to reduce the probability that the abuse or neglect will recur, causing more head injury.

4
Psychiatric and Behavioral Disorders of Children

Just as specific focal signs are less common in neurological disorders of children than they are in adults, so too specific, discrete psychiatric symptoms are less common in children with psychiatric disorders than in adults. The most common symptoms of childhood psychiatric disorders are aggressiveness, acting out, impulsivity, and antisocial behavior. Children with different psychiatric or behavioral disorders may show combinations of these symptoms in varying permutations. Often, neurological abnormalities are associated with the behavioral disorders. On the other hand, children with neurological disorders and symptoms are at greater risk to develop behavioral disorders than are children without neurological disorders.

Current theories and research studies in the neuropsychology of childhood psychiatric disorders agree in the observed association between neuropsychological impairment and behavioral or emotional disturbances, but disagree as to the exact relationship. Are the psychiatric symptoms the direct result of the brain dysfunction causing the neuropsychological impairments? Are the behavioral and emotional problems secondary to greater difficulty in functioning experienced by the neuropsychologically impaired child? Regardless of the exact relationship, the connection between these two types of problems indicates that the child clinician should be sensitive to the possible presence of neuropsychological difficulties in the child who presents with behavioral abnormalities and to the possible presence of behavioral and emotional difficulties in the child who presents with a neurological disorder.

The relationships between the two types of disorders and symptoms is complex and cannot be dealt with sufficiently in a chapter of this nature. However, this chapter will review some of the observed relations to alert the clinician to the possibilities. Although it was originally thought that the degree of neuropsychological impairment was related to the level of emotional disturbance, there is evidence to suggest that this is too simplistic of a description (Dean, 1986). Although the DSM-III R contains categories for mental retardation and other developmental disorders, those disorders will not be discussed in this chapter but rather in the chapter on disorders of delayed development.

CONDUCT DISORDERS

Some of the most common psychiatric diagnoses for children involve behavior that is aggressive or otherwise unsocialized. These children may resort to physical force to effect their desires more frequently than nondisordered children, or they may engage in seemingly purposeless aggression. There is evidence to suggest that many of these children exhibit neuropsychological problems such as impulsivity, poor abstract problem-solving skills, or deficient academic achievement. Frequently unsocialized behavior will be seen in a child with a history of a head injury. Socialization occurs as the result of observational and contingent learning on the part of the child. Children who are raised in a household where physical means are often used to settle disputes or in an environment of inconsistent contingencies may exhibit conduct disorders without accompanying neuropsychological signs.

CHILDHOOD SCHIZOPHRENIA

Children may exhibit psychotic symptoms due to situational stress. The symptoms may occur on a transient basis. Children with schizophrenia additionally will exhibit thought disorders. As the child grows older, the symptoms will more closely approximate the symptoms of adult schizophrenia. Childhood schizophrenia is associated with various developmental delays, including delays in the age when the child first walks and talks. They may also show problems in integration of sensory, motor, and perceptual functions and difficulty in sustaining attention. Children who show these delays can be monitored for the later appearance of the symptoms of schizophrenia. Later signs of poor academic achievement, deficient abstract problem-solving skills, and abnormal language use may also occur.

AFFECTIVE DISORDERS

Major affective disorders have a genetic component that suggests an organic etiology. However, in these cases there is usually not a systematic relation-

Psychiatric and Behavioral Disorders of Children

ship between the affective disorder and symptoms of neuropsychological impairment. These children may show poor academic achievement secondary to the affective symptoms rather than to an organic etiology. Often a depressive disorder is paradoxically manifested in a child by increased levels of activity and aggressive behavior. Psychiatric and psychological intervention can be effective in treating these disorders.

ANXIETY DISORDERS

Anxiety is a common symptom in children with psychiatric disorders. In cases where anxiety is the cardinal feature, an emotional disorder such as separation anxiety, avoidant disorder, or overanxious disorder may be diagnosed. Although there does not appear to be a central nervous system etiology for these disorders, there may be neuropsychological symptoms secondary to the emotional disorder. The anxiety may decrease the attention span of the child, causing poor performance on those tasks requiring sustained attention. Here the level of performance on attentional tasks will vary with the degree of anxious symptoms experienced by the child. Novel situations or persons will exacerbate the difficulties. Habituation to the situation or adequate treatment of the anxious symptoms should decrease the attentional problems.

EATING DISORDERS

Eating disorders can result in neuropsychological difficulties. Anorexia can cause nutritional deficiencies resulting in lowered levels of neuropsychological skill. Bulimia when accompanied by induced vomiting may result in electrolyte imbalances and lowered abstraction skills, poor higher order integration skills, and lowered concentration and attention. All of these may first be noticed when academic achievement suffers. In small children, a rumination disorder may impact on developmental level by causing nutritional deficiencies. Pica may cause neuropsychological deficits secondary to ingestion of neurotoxins.

INFANTILE AUTISM

Infantile autism is ususally diagnosed before the age of 30 months. The hallmarks of infantile autism include failure to develop social relationships, retarded development of communication skills, and compulsive behaviors. Autistic children may exhibit *echolalia*, or repetition of spoken communications. Clinical lore states that these children are intellectually bright, but empirical evidence suggests that there may be intellectual retardation in the presence of adequate visual spatial skills (DeMyer, 1975).

Other disorders of childhood, although not commonly thought of as psychiatric disorders, are often diagnosed and treated by child psychiatrists. They are included in the DSM-III R and are therefore contained in this chapter. These include attention deficit disorders and learning disabilities.

ATTENTION DEFICIT DISORDER

There are two general forms of Attention Deficit Disorder (ADD): with and without hyperactivity. In both cases, the central features are shortened attention span, impulsivity, and distractibility. When high levels of activity are included, the diagnosis is amended to ADD with hyperactivity. Children with this disorder show pervasive deficits in attention and in rule-governed behavior, but these deficits are not due to impairment in sensory or perceptual functions, motor activity or skills, other psychiatric disorders, neurological disorders, or mental retardation. Generally, these children (mainly boys) have near-average IQ, but academic achievement is limited by the attentional deficits.

As might be deduced from the name, the cardinal neuropsychological feature of these two disorders is a deficit in attention processes. Neuropsychological tests that require sustained attention or that penalize impulsive performance will classify these children as impaired. However, if the child can be induced to attend, usually in a one-to-one setting, adequate achievement can be demonstrated.

There have been many theories regarding the etiology of ADD. Early theories postulated that ADD was secondary to brain damage, mainly because the symptom of hyperactivity is often seen following brain damage, particularly postencephalitis. However, there have not been any data documenting the presence of structural brain damage in ADD. Congenital etiologies were also proposed, but again, there has been no subsequent unequivocal empirical evidence.

Recently, there has been much focus in the popular media regarding a purported relationship between food additives and hyperactivity or between sugar and hyperactivity, but again, systematic empirical evidence is lacking. Stamm and Kreder (1979) have proposed a theory that ADD may be the result of late maturation of the frontal lobes, a notion supported by Connors (Connors & Wells, 1986). The evidence for this theory, although attractive, is inferential. Yet another set of theories posits a biochemical dysfunction. Evidence for these theories is taken largely from the effect of psychoactive drugs in the treatment of ADD.

Optimal treatment of ADD involves some combination of central nervous system stimulants and behavioral management strategies. The medication seems to improve the attention span, and the behavioral treatment seems to increase compliance and academic achievement. A complete neuropsychological evaluation may be helpful in planning treatment or education approaches in children with ADD.

DEVELOPMENTAL MOTOR DISORDERS

The DSM III-R recognizes the existence of disorders that present primarily as impaired motor coordination. These conditions may sometimes be due to a neurological disorder, and in those cases, the DSM III-R diagnosis of Developmental Coordination Disorder cannot be given. In these children there is a marked delay in the development of the ability to perform coordinated motor activities such as tieing their shoes, playing sports, or other behaviors that require fine motor coordination such as printing. The children may have been labelled as clumsy. These disorders are not secondary to mental retardation or a neurological disorder. Often they are associated with delays in other developmental skills.

LEARNING DISORDERS

In the legal arena, learning disorders are diagnosed on the basis of average IQ but subaverage academic achievement in some area. Specific learning disabilities may occur in the areas of arithmetic, reading, spelling, or writing. These children are in need of early intervention to help avoid later adjustment and vocational problems. A history of failure experiences can engender poor self-image and affective symptoms.

Under DSM III-R, children with learning disabilities are often given diagnoses of Academic Skills Disorders. The criteria for the DSM III-R diagnoses do not require that IQ values be in the average range. Instead, the diagnoses require that the academic achievement of the child as measured by standardized achievement tests be inconsistent with the IQ values obtained from an individually administered IQ test. Therefore, it is possible that a child may receive a DSM III-R diagnosis without being legally eligible for specialized school services. The clinician should keep this in mind and should also be prepared to explain to parents why their child has been given a diagnosis but is still not eligible for services. In these cases, the child clinician can act as an ombudsman for the child, working with the school system to help provide appropriate teaching services inside the structure determined by the available resources. The DSM III-R diagnoses under

Academic Skills Disorders include Developmental Arithmetic Disorder, Developmental Expressive Writing Disorder, and Developmental Reading Disorder.

Reading disabilities are known as dyslexia, although the term dyslexias would be more accurate. There have been many theories on the etiology of dyslexia, the most well known of which is the left hemisphere lesion theory or abnormal hemispheric asymmetry theory (Orton, 1937). This theory has been debunked, but has not been replaced by any single theory. The diversity of theories is probably due to the fact that many different subskills compose adequate reading skills and dysfunction of any one of them can cause dyslexia. Classic dyslexia is perceptual, in which the child reverses letters. Other forms of dyslexia may be secondary to deficits in successive or simultaneous processing, deficits in understanding morpheme–phoneme relationships, or difficulty in combining letters into words.

Other subtypes of learning disabilities are possible and probably represent an even richer mix of etiologies and manifestations. It is important to remember that failure to achieve in a given academic area may be related to environmental as well as to organic factors. Organic impairment should not be assumed in learning disabled children, but observed relationships between some learning disabilities and some forms of neuropsychological deficits indicate the need to assess each child independently.

DISORDERS NOT OTHERWISE SPECIFIED

A final DSM III-R category is that of Specific Developmental Disorder Not Otherwise Specified (NOS). Specific developmental disorders, that is, disorders in the development of academic skills, motor skills, or language skills that do not fit the descriptions given for their related DSM III-R diagnoses may require a diagnosis of Specific Developmental Disorder NOS. However, if the child exhibits a more widespread pattern of developmental delays, the diagnosis of Pervasive Developmental Disorder may instead be appropriate.

5
Neurological Soft Signs

The term *soft signs* was developed in contrast to neurological *hard signs.* Therefore, a discussion of both terms is necessary to the understanding of either. A hard sign can be thought of as a pathognomonic sign. Hard signs are symptoms of neurobehavioral disturbance and are often associated with a particular disorder of the central nervous system. For example, abnormalities of pupillary reflexes are considered to be hard signs, as are hemiplegia, aphasia, and constructional dyspraxias.

Soft signs can be thought of as behavioral symptoms that are related probabilistically to disorders of the central nervous system. Soft signs are not always accompanied by disorders of the central nervous system and do not have a relationship to any particular disorder. Examples of soft signs in children include associated movements (lesser movements in another part of the body that accompany purposeful movement), motor awkwardness, and lateness in reaching developmental milestones.

There is a wider range of signs considered to be "soft" for children than there is for adults, because of the greater variability of behavioral performance in children. Not all children reach developmental milestones at the same age, although extremely late demonstration of milestone behaviors is certainly a cause for concern. In younger children, use of telegraphic speech will raise concerns but will not be the diagnostic indicator that this phenomenon is for older children and adults.

This raises an important issue. Many soft signs in children are actually the demonstration of lateness in reaching milestones or in suppressing infantile reflexes. Therefore it is extremely important to always be comparing the performance of the child to developmental norms. In those cases where the clinician can follow a child over time, the acquisition of milestones can be monitored and increasing developmental delays can alert the general clinician to the need for referral to a specialist.

THE CONTROVERSY RELATED TO SOFT SIGNS

The measurement of soft signs is somewhat controversial. The controversy, which is partly related to the nascent state of standardization in this area, is fueled by considerations of the tradition from which the concept of soft signs developed. In children, the concept of soft signs is related to the concept of minimal brain dysfunction (MBD). It is no understatement to suggest that MBD is not a universally accepted notion. The brain dysfunction in MBD is assumed. Although there is more rationality associated with the diagnosis of MBD currently, earlier uses of the diagnostic term tended to be overly inclusive. MBD was assumed when a child demonstrated difficulty in academic areas or late development without objective signs of central nervous dysfunction such as abnormal computed tomography (CT) results or EEG records. Unfortunately, this assumption engendered problems because it did not consider the environmental influences on performance of developmental and academic tasks.

The use of soft signs in diagnosis is often criticized because of the large amount of heterogeneity in their behavioral manifestations. Tupper (1986) suggests that soft signs be divided into at least two subcategories, developmental soft signs and soft signs of abnormality. Developmental soft signs are signs that the child has not reached developmental milestones at the usual time. Soft signs of abnormality are those signs that would be considered abnormal regardless of the age of the child. By proposing this distinction, Tupper hopes to reduce some of the confusion regarding the measurement of soft signs.

There is a body of evidence that suggests that soft signs are associated with learning disabilities, hyperactivity, and minimal brain dysfunction. The list of associated disorders points out some of the problems in using soft signs as diagnostic indicators. Many of these disorders have not been conclusively shown to be the result of brain impairment. However, it should be pointed out that soft signs are also associated with some forms of demonstrated neuropathology (Touwen, 1987).

There are other considerations regarding the acceptance of soft signs. For one, soft signs are often criticized for their lack of reliability. Soft signs are thought to lack interrater as well as temporal reliability. However, it is important to separate the phenomenological concept from the measurement system. It is not the soft signs that lack acceptable reliability, but rather the method of measurement. The clinical-behavioral literature has many examples of measurement systems that have been developed to allow the reliable measurement of behavior. There is no reason to believe that the same cannot be done for soft signs, which are, after all, behaviors. Unfortunately, this has not been accomplished as yet, despite recent advances in the area.

An important consideration in the measurement of soft signs is the issue of validity. In neuropsychological assessment, validation is partly accomplished by comparison of the results of the neuropsychological assessment to the results of objective neurodiagnostic methods such as angiography and CT scans. Due to the nature of soft signs, this system is not appropriate for validating soft signs. Soft signs are subtle indications of supposed central nervous system dysfunction. Their utility is increased to the extent that they can predict the later occurrence of objective signs of dysfunction. Predictive validation endeavors therefore acquire a greater importance than concurrent validation endeavors in the case of soft signs.

Another consideration of validity involves an examination of the purposes to which the measurement of soft signs is put. It is important to remember that tests are not validated; rather, inferences drawn from test results are validated. At this point it is safe to conclude that the measurement of soft signs should not be used to diagnose specific disorders. However, the measurement of soft signs can be useful in the prediction of later objective dysfunction or in the decision to refer to a specialist for a more complete evaluation.

RELATIONSHIP OF SOFT SIGNS TO NEUROLOGICAL DISORDERS

Part of the attraction of soft signs is undoubtedly their relationship to disorders that are assumed to be neurological in basis but for which few clear hard signs are reliably found. There is greater interest in these disorders in children than in adults. In addition, it is more difficult to devise assessment instruments for children than it is for adults. Adults have a wider range of skills to be evaluated through an assessment instrument. As little as we really know about adult brain–behavior relationships, child brain–behavior relationships are even less well understood. There is a wider range of variability in child cortico-behavioral manifestations as the child is in a greater state of flux than the adult.

All of these conditions and factors combine to create a situation where measurement of qualitative aspects of behavior has a potentially greater importance for children. In the relative absence of definite hard signs, assessment of the soft signs acquires greater emphasis. Even though there are observed relationships between the presence of soft signs and the concurrent diagnoses of disorders assumed to have a central nervous system etiology, it is important to remember the limitations on the interpretation of these soft signs. First, the presence of the soft signs does not always denote the concurrent presence of a particular diagnosis. Soft signs tend to be nonspecific referents of neurological disorders and may be present in children who do not have a disorder with a central nervous system etiology. Second, the association of soft signs with a given disorder does not prove that the particular disorder has a central nervous system etiology. With those limitations in mind, let us review some of the disorders that have been found to be associated with soft signs.

DISORDERS ASSOCIATED WITH SOFT SIGNS

Our understanding of the neurological effects of pregnancy and birth complications is limited by a dearth of longitudinal studies following the development of children who experience these complications. The obstetrician who is aware of the complications does not follow the infant once born, and the pediatric neurologist who does follow the infant may not have a complete understanding of the complications. However, it does appear that children who experience hypoxic events show a greater frequency of soft signs which may be secondary to brain damage engendered by the hypoxic events. Hypoxia can occur either prenatally or perinatally. The situation is complicated further by the fact that perinatal hypoxic events may be the result of prenatal damage to brain areas responsible for respiratory functions. For example, *apnea,* or a sudden, usually brief arrest of respiratory function, is not uncommon in infants and may be related to sudden infant death. The associated soft signs may be related to the effects of the hypoxic state secondary to the apnea or to the original brain lesion that was responsible for the apnea. Regardless of the causal relationships with the soft signs, hypoxic events in pregnancy and early life may be due to dysfunction of the placenta, crimping of the umbilical cord, maternal illness, premature birth, or physical injury.

There have been many criticisms of studies that attempt to investigate the relationship between soft signs and psychiatric diagnosis. Aspects of the studies considered to be shortcomings range from the use of biased samples to use of insufficiently defined diagnostic or heterogeneous groups (Shaffer, O'Connor, Shafer, & Prupis 1983). Because the relationship is poorly understood, it best to describe it as probabilistic—that children with psychiatric disorder tend to exhibit a greater frequency of soft signs. It may be that a dysfunction of the central nervous system is directly responsible for both the soft signs and the psychiatric disorder. Alternatively, it is possible that the soft signs represent some central nervous system dysfunction that causes difficulty in adjustment, resulting in the behavioral manifestations of psychiatric disorders. Or it may be that developmental delays not related to central nervous system lesions are more common in children with psychiatric disorders.

Hyperactivity, or in the nomenclature of DSM-III R, attention deficit disorder with hyperactivity, is actually diagnosed on the basis of behavioral observations. Evidence for the assumed central nervous system etiology of hyperactive behavior is found in the presence of soft signs with these children and in the response of many of these children to psychoactive medication. It has already been noted that soft signs cannot be seen as strong evidence for central nervous system disorders. It is also dangerous to assume that because psychoactive drugs reduce the symptoms of a disorder, the symptoms are due to a central nervous system dysfunction "corrected" by the drugs. Attention deficit disorder (ADD) may also be seen in children who do not exhibit hyperactivity, further detracting from conclusions regarding a single central nervous system dysfunction.

The core symptoms of ADD are a short attention span, distractibility and impulsivity. Children with ADD are more likely to exhibit a greater frequency of soft signs and neurological abnormalities. With the possible exceptions of a greater frequency of associated movements (synkinesia) and less skilled fine motor function, there does not appear to be any regularity in the type of soft sign exhibited by these children. It should be noted that in one study, associated movements were found in only 28% of the children with a diagnosis of ADD (Levine, Busch, & Aufseeser, 1982).

Learning disabilities are defined as deficient achievement in one or more academic areas that are not the result of mental retardation, emotional disorders, environmental deprivation, motor disabilities, or sensory disorders. Learning disorders may be secondary to perceptual disorders. Children with a specific learning disorder will show adequate achievement in other academic areas. Although learning disabled children are more likely to show soft signs, there does not appear to be a characteristic syndrome of soft signs associated with learning disabilities. This may be due to the usually heterogeneous grouping of learning disabled children in these studies or to a lack of a direct relationship between the soft signs and the learning disability. However, because of the possibility that soft signs in a learning disabled child may reflect a central nervous system dysfunction, learning disabled children who exhibit soft signs should probably be referred for evaluation by a specialist.

CLASSIFICATION AND ASSESSMENT OF SOFT SIGNS

Although the original use of the term "soft signs" was to differentiate them from neurological hard signs, the detection of a soft sign should still require objective evidence. There should be little question as to the presence of the sign. The hard/soft distinction refers to the degree of relationship between the sign and the presence of an underlying neurological disorder. Soft signs occur in individuals in whom there are no hard or pathognomonic signs of central nervous system dysfunction. In fact, the only evidence for central nervous system dysfunction in these individuals may be the presence of soft signs and lack of appropriate academic achievement or behavioral adjustment difficulties.

Tupper (1986) has listed some possible soft signs designated as either developmental soft signs or soft signs of abnormality. Developmental soft signs are those behavioral signs that are abnormal only because they are age-inappropriate. Soft signs of abnormality are behaviors that would be abnormal, largely independent of the age of the child. We will first consider the developmental soft signs. Although it is possible for any developmental delay to be seen as a soft sign, Tupper has indicated that some delays are more serious than others.

Developmental Soft Signs

There are two general forms of developmental soft signs. The first form involves behavioral signs exhibited by a child beyond the age at which most children have outgrown the behavior. An example of this type of developmental soft sign is motor awkwardness, which would be expected in very young children but not in older children. Motor awkwardness would be considered a soft sign only for older children. The second type of developmental soft sign is a behavior that is not exhibited by a child when most children of the same age can be expected to exhibit it. For example, a child who does not begin to walk by the age of two years shows this kind of developmental soft sign.

One of the most serious developmental soft signs is the presence of associated movements. Associated movements, sometimes known as overflow or mirror movements, are seen when the child engages in a purposeful movement of a limb and mirrors that movement to a lesser extent in another limb. For example, in touching his fingers one at a time to his thumb on his right hand, the child will involuntarily make minimal movements with his left hand that resemble the movement of the right hand. This is sometimes known by the term *synkinesis.* The clinician can observe for this phenomenon during the interview and evaluation or she may try to elicit the behavior by asking the child to perform some movements with one limb while keeping the other limb still.

Other developmental soft signs discussed by Tupper (1986) include difficulty in building with blocks, immature grasp of a pencil, and inability to catch a ball. Although each of these behaviors can be associated with developmental delays, it is important to note that each is also partly under the control of environmental variables such as the amount of experience with the behavior. For example, a child with an older sibling who engages the young child in ball games is likely to learn to catch a ball before a child without access to such experience. Difficulty in building with blocks changes at different age levels. Immature grasp of a pencil may be influenced to a lesser degree by experience, but even here, there may be variability in the age at which a child acquires a mature grasp, usually by three years.

Lateness in meeting developmental milestones and in suppressing primitive reflexes is also on Tupper's list. Lateness in suppressing primitive reflexes is best evaluated by a pediatric neurologist. Yet another developmental soft sign discussed by Tupper is motor awkwardness or clumsiness for age. Unfortunately, assessing whether or not a child is clumsy for his age requires some subjectivity in evaluating the observations. The observations of the clinician can be combined with statements from parents and teachers regarding the motor behavior of the child in comparison to his peers and siblings. Two frequently used methods of assessing clumsiness are to ask the child either to tap his finger and thumb together or to tap successive fingers to this thumb. The relevant score is the number of accurate taps in a given period of time. Poor performance can be the result of deficits in motor activity or in visual judgment of distance and direction.

Motor impersistence is a loosely defined concept. However, we are fortunate in that Benton has provided standardized instructions and age-related norms for several behavioral tasks of motor impersistence. In Benton, Hamsher, Varney, & Spreen (1983) a standardized test called the Test of Motor Impersistence is described, and the results of administering the test to 140 normal children between the ages of 5 and 11 years are reported. The test consists of eight tasks: keeping one's eyes shut, protruding one's tongue (eyes closed), protruding one's tongue (eyes open), fixation of gaze in lateral visual fields, keeping one's mouth open, central fixation during confrontation testing of visual fields, head turning during sensory testing, and saying "ah." The tasks are described to the child, who is then asked to perform the behavior as long as possible while the clinician times the procedures. Scoring is on the basis of how many of the tasks are failed compared to the normative sample.

The gait and posture of the child also play a role in the detection of developmental soft signs. Poor gait, posture, or stance can be suggestive of a soft sign. It is important for the clinician to determine the extent to which the child can assume correct posture and the extent to which the child demonstrates correct posture consistently. Particularly important would be the exhibition of asymmetric posture. Other soft signs include slow gait or slow hand movements or fingertapping.

The presence of difficulty in speech articulation can be a soft sign. However, it should be pointed out that many children have poor articulation even late into life without any associated signs of organic impairment. As with any of the soft signs, the presence of one such soft sign is insufficient to necessitate a diagnosis. However, the presence of two or more coupled with evidence of academic difficulties may be enough evidence to suggest that referral to a specialist is in order.

The final soft sign is tactile extinction on double simultaneous stimulation. To evaluate for the presence of this symptom, the clinician first asks the child to close her eyes or else a blindfold is placed on the child's head. Using a cotton swab or wadded tissue, the clinician then touches first the back of one hand and then the back of the child's other hand, asking the child to identify which hand is being touched. Be sure that the touch is gentle and only firm enough to be registered by the child. After a few random touches to either hand, the clinician then without warning touches the back of both hands and repeats the cycle. If the child can consistently identify the correct hand when one hand at a time is touched but cannot identify when both hands are touched at the same time, what is known as *suppression* has occurred. This is a fairly strong sign of central nervous system dysfunction.

Soft Signs of Abnormality

The soft signs of abnormality are behavioral anomalies that would be considered abnormal regardless of the age at which they appear. They are still less diagnostic than are hard signs. These soft signs of abnormality would also be a reason for concern if they occurred in adults.

Some of the soft signs of abnormality are best evaluated by a neurologist. These include diffuse EEG abnormalities, pathological reflexes, reflex asymmetries, increases or decreases of the reflex from normal, and increases or decreases in normal muscle tone. Other of these signs are as easily evaluated by a general child clinician as by a specialist.

The signs for which a general child clinician is able to assess include *astereognosis*. Astereognosis is an impairment in the ability to recognize an object from the sense of touch alone without using sight, smell, or taste. To evaluate for this abnormality, the clinician can blindfold the patient and then place simple common objects in one hand at a time, asking the patient to identify the objects. These objects can include a coin (ask for the exact type of coin handed to the patient), a button, a thimble, or a safety pin. The subject should be allowed to feel the object only with one hand at a time, and the procedure should be timed. Most children over the age of nine years should be able to identify each object within 20 seconds or less. It is important to state here that if the patient can identify the object by describing its use but cannot produce its name, a problem other than astereognosis is present, namely word-finding difficulty. However, word-finding difficulty is also a soft sign of abnormality.

Word-finding difficulty can also be assessed during the interview and throughout the evaluation. If the patient exhibits tip of the tongue phenomenon consistently, then word-finding difficulty may be present. Another method of assessing for this soft sign is to present pictures of everyday objects and ask the patient to name them. Consistent failure to do so in the presence of an ability to describe their uses is evidence of word-finding difficulty. Other language abnormalities that can be assessed during the interview include *dysarthria,* or incorrect pronunciation. Here, the clinician needs to evaluate the pronunciation of the patient against the local norms and the developmental norms. This is relatively easy to do if the child comes from the same geographical area as does the clinician. If the clinician or the child's family has recently moved to the locale where the evaluation takes place, greater sensitivity of the clinician to idiosyncratic pronunciation is required.

Dysgraphesthesia is the inability to identify numbers or letters written on the skin of the patient while the patient is blindfolded. The clinician can keep a stylus in his office to test this ability. Or, alternately, a ballpoint pen that has run out of ink might be used.

Some motor signs are also considered by Tupper (1986) to be soft signs of abnormality. These include *hypokinesis* (or lowered levels of motor activity), choreiform movements (or sudden, asymmetric purposeless movements), oromotor apraxia, drooling, nystagmus (spasmodic movement of the eyes), tremor, posturing of hands while walking, and significant incoordination. Unfortunately, not all of these signs are well defined behaviorally.

Choreiform movements are perhaps the most readily noticeable of this class of motor signs. Sometimes it may be necessary to ask the child to engage in a simple behavior such as raising her hands above her head to elicit the choreiform movements. The choreiform movement is noticed when the fingers are extended, not when they are still in motion. *Tremor* is subtle shakiness of body parts. It may be of two types. An intentional tremor occurs only when the child attempts to initiate movement. An at rest tremor occurs when movement is absent and disappears when the child attempts movement.

The clinician wishing to perform a more rigorous evaluation for the presence of soft signs can use one of the structured instruments. (See Tupper 1987 for details). It should be noted that the utility of these structured instruments has not been decisively determined. However, the clinician might find them useful in helping to alert himself to the presence of any of the soft signs. As noted above, the presence of soft signs should not be interpreted diagnostically, but the presence of several of the soft signs may be seen as sufficient reason for referral to a specialist.

NEUROLOGICAL DYSFUNCTION OF CHILDREN

In its manual, the Neurological Dysfunction of Children (NDOC) (Kuhns, 1979) is described as being applicable to children between the ages of 3 and 10 years. It has a somewhat limited scope in that it was designed to identify children who have a neurologically based learning disorder. To the extent that a clinician's practice is largely composed of children who might have learning disorders or who are referred for evaluation because of academic difficulties, the NDOC can be very useful. The behaviors elicited in the NDOC are broad based, but the interpretation suggestions found in the manual are limited to subtypes of learning disorders. Clinicians who work in a medical setting or who have occasion to see children for reasons other than academic difficulties may not find the NDOC useful unless they are familiar enough with neurodevelopmental theory to use the procedures to guide their own assessment procedures but use a more general interpretation strategy.

A strength of the NDOC is that it can be used by school psychologists, child clinical psychologists, and physicians. Another strength of the NDOC is its brevity. As part of the NDOC, the child is asked to perform 16 behaviors such as walking along a straight line, walking on tiptoe, walking on heels, visual fixation, visual pursuit, and tongue movements. The seventeenth item is measurement of the head circumference of the child, and the eighteenth item is a structured interview with the parents to obtain a developmental history.

The scoring system of the NDOC is reported in the manual as being highly reliable; however, this is based on a sample of only 19 children between the ages of 3 and 12 years. In addition, all of the children in the reliability study were recruited from a university laboratory school and were reported to be functioning in the normal range. Given the setting from which the children were recruited, it is more likely that they were functioning in the above-average range. Be that as it may, the children were not likely to fail many of the items. The more important but unaddressed question asks about the reliability of the test in an impaired sample.

The NDOC is scored on a binary basis (pass or fail) for each of the items on the basis of developmental norms by age. The item scores are then grouped into 13 clusters, and referral for further evaluation is suggested depending on which cluster the child's performance approximates. Interpretation of the clusters and of each of the items is described in the manual. It should be noted that of the two validity studies reported in the manual, neither is methodologically adequate. The NDOC can therefore be recommended for use only as a method to organize one's observations. The interpretation strategies from the manual are best ignored by the clinician who is not familiar with neurobehavioral theory. Instead the general child clinician should report the results to the referral specialist in the form of which behaviors the child was and was not able to perform.

PHYSICAL AND NEUROLOGICAL EXAMINATION FOR SOFT SIGNS

The Physical and Neurological Examination for Soft Signs (PANESS) (Guy, 1976) is administered on the basis of a four-page protocol describing the procedures used. In addition, there is a 12-page manual describing the administration of the neurological examination designed by John Close. The PANESS was originally developed at the National Institute of Mental Health, from which the protocol is available. It was developed as part of a drug evaluation study but is now used in a variety of settings. The PANESS may be the most commonly used standardized assessment instrument for the evaluation of soft signs in children. The first part of the PANESS involves a physical examination of the child and its administration is therefore limited to physicians. This part of the PANESS requires evaluation of the age, weight, height, pulse, blood pressure, and visual acuity; evaluation of liver, kidney, and spleen function; and assessment of musculoskeletal, gross neurological, and lymphatic status.

The second part of the PANESS is an evaluation for behavioral soft signs and is appropriate for use by other child clinicians. The procedures involve asking the child to perform finger-to-nose movements with eyes open and closed, and analogous heel-to-shin movements. Next, the child is asked to identify or draw objects that the clinician has drawn on her hand while the child was blindfolded. Walking on tiptoe, walking on heels, hopping on one foot, and walking heel to toe forward and backward make up the next part of the PANESS. The subsequent section involves simultaneous stimulation, motor persistence procedures, and timed finger and foot tapping. Finally, visual pursuit is tested.

The PANESS has the advantage of possessing scoring criteria for four different levels of performance, resulting in acquisition of more information than would be obtained simply by scoring in a binary fashion. Reliability of the PANESS has been evaluated and found to be adequate, but failure on many of the items may be low rate occurrences, somewhat limiting the diagnostic utility of the instrument.

Quick Neurological Screening Test

The Quick Neurological Screening Test (QNST) (Mutti, Sterling, & Spalding, 1978) is a short evaluation of soft signs that can be administered in 10 to 15 minutes. It can be administered by general child clinicians. There are a total of 15 items that test many of the functions that should be familiar to the reader by now. These procedures include tandem walking, finger-to-nose movements, double simultaneous stimulation, visual tracking, figure recognition and reproduction, and hand skill. Both numerical quantitative scores and qualitative scores are possible, but the reliability of the individual items ranges from 0.93 for the Hand Preference Test to 0.43 for the Eye Preference Test. The manual includes a number of interpretative considerations. The major focus of the QNST is the identification of children who will experience trouble in academic tasks. Therefore, the test might be better called the Quick Learning Disability Screening Test (Rattan & Dean, 1985). Despite the limitations, the QNST might be useful in identifying children for whom a more rigorous evaluation is necessary.

OVERVIEW

The methodology in the assessment of neurological soft signs has shown great improvement in recent times. Earlier criticisms of nonstandardized administration and scoring have been met with more rigorous protocols. However, some of the conceptual criticisms of the meaning of the soft signs may still hold. It is probably best to view the soft signs as indicators of the need for a more specialized evaluation, and as such, standardized evaluations of soft signs may present useful procedures for the general child clinician wishing to decide whether to refer to a specialist. Interpretation of soft signs is best limited to rudimentary considerations. The general child clinicians might instead wish to limit the information in her report to descriptions of the behavioral signs observed.

Part II
EVALUATING THE CHILD

6
The Interview and History

The clinical interview can be a rich source of information regarding the need to refer to a specialist for a more complete evaluation. The clinician can obtain objective information regarding the particulars of the presenting complaint, the clinical history of the child, and the relationship of the child to others in the environment. By careful observation, the clinician can also obtain information regarding the child–parent interaction, the presence of qualitative speech problems, the presence of abnormal motor activity, and the level of affective functioning.

The clinical interview itself can be seen as a screening device. It is here that the clinician can begin to gain an understanding of what the problem is (diagnosis) as well as what seems to be causing the problem (etiology). During the interview, the clinician obtains information that can be helpful in choosing tests to administer to the child. Also during the interview, the clinician can start generating hypotheses that later can be tested against data obtained from other sources.

INTERVIEWING THE CHILD

Interviewing the child requires specific techniques that are particular to this population. Of course, interviewing a child also requires some of the same considerations taken in interviewing an adult, such as demonstrating an attitude of respect, developing a mutually trusting interaction style, objectively evaluating the patient's statements without dismissing them out of hand, using open-ended questions to elicit more information, and structuring the interview to maximize the efficiency with which information is acquired.

The aspects of interviewing that are unique to working with children involve gearing the language to the developmental and intellectual level of the child and making allowances for the child's attitude toward the clinician (Simmons, 1987). It is important to keep in mind that the behavior of children may be under more strict control by social environmental variables than that of adults. Another important difference between adults and children in psychological and psychiatric evaluations is that the child is invariably brought in by another individual. In that sense, interviewing a child is somewhat similar to interviewing an adult for forensic purposes or for the purpose of commitment. The clinician must make an extra effort to enlist the cooperation and trust of the child.

For these reasons it is extremely important to determine the child's understanding of the reasons for referral and evaluation. The child may only know that he is being brought there because he "did something." In the child's mind, the evaluation may be tantamount to punishment for failure to produce academic achievement or failure to behave. The child's only previous experience with a doctor may have involved painful hypodermic needles or cold stethoscopes. To the extent that the child can understand the reason for referral, the clinician should communicate the reason as honestly as possibly. Children may appear to be naive, but they are usually very perceptive in detecting false assurances or hypocrisy in adults.

Speaking frankly but gently with the child can help engender a cooperative context for the evaluation. For example, the clinician might first ask the child why he thinks he was brought to the evaluation and what he was told regarding what would take place in the interview. Then the clinician may respond with "Your parents and teachers asked me to see you so I could help you find out why you're having trouble in school. I'll be asking you some questions. Some of the questions will be about your feelings. Some questions will be about how you think." If during the interview or evaluation, the child shows signs of discomfort over the difficulty of the tests, the clinician can state, "I know that some of these questions will be hard for you and some will be easy. Just do the best that you can."

The child often senses that prior communication between the parents and the clinician has occurred. The clinician can minimize the effects of this suspicion by stating outright that the parents already said that "You were having trouble in spelling, even though you are doing okay in arithmetic," or "Your parents already told me that you have a hard time sitting still in class. What do you think?"

The clinician is well advised to structure the situation so that equal considerations are given to the child and the parents. One method of doing this is to briefly interview the child with the parents first, then interview the child alone, then interview the parents alone, and finally have a brief closing interview with the child. This structure should be explained to the child ahead of time. Telling the child that he will get a period of time with the clinician—just as the parents will—helps communicate to the child that he and his information are viewed as being as important as the parents and their information.

Interviewing the child together with the parents has the added benefit of allowing observations of a sample of the parent–child interaction patterns. Seeing the child alone a second time gives the child a chance to have the last word and allows the clinician an opportunity to follow-up on additional information provided by the parents in their interview. For very young children (under the age of two years), a solitary interview may not be possible because of fretfulness of the child when the mother is not present.

Of course, observing the parent–child interaction during the interview may provide a limited and somewhat biased sample due to the novelty of the situation (Gross, 1985). Therefore, the parents should be asked to what extent the behavior of the child during the joint interview was different from her usual behavior. Similarly, the child can be asked to describe the extent to which the interview behavior of the parents differed from their usual behavior. Both the child and the parents should be instructed to provide information as honestly and openly as possible. Although this cannot ensure that honesty and openness will prevail, the instructions can increase that probability, thereby enhancing the efficiency of the interview time.

Observing the differences in behavior of the child with the parents and alone may provide useful information. On more than one occasion, we have seen children who when with their parents did not answer the clinician's questions, but would instead look at them, waiting for one to respond. Quick responses by the parents were often followed by willingness of the child to talk in the solitary interview. In this case the observed behavior would probably be the result of interactional variables between the child and parents rather than of language difficulties of the child.

The use of language presents special problems for the child clinician. Younger children do not effectively use or well understand abstract communication. Even if the child uses language constructions that imply abstractions, the clinician's communication should be fairly concrete. The clinician should ask for clarifications of any of the child's language that appears to be abstract. The child may be only parroting verbalizations without fully comprehending the symbolic referents. For older children and adolescents, the clinician needs to be conversant with the contemporary lingo. Although there are similarities of slang in a single age group, there are also differences across neighborhoods, schools, or even peer groups. The clinician should ask for clarification while avoiding sounding like another adult "idiot." A fair rule of thumb is that if the clinician is having trouble understanding the colloquialisms of the child, the child is similarly having difficulty understanding the adult verbal constructions of the clinician.

Many children have learned to say, "I don't know" when in fact they mean, "I don't want to discuss it." In our culture, a child is expected always to answer an adult's questions as part of the "respect your elders" dictum. Adult authority figures may demand answers to their questions and may not allow attempts by the child to decline comment. As part of developing a trusting relationship with the child, the clinician can give permission to say, "I don't want to talk about it right now." This gives the child a chance to exert some autonomy and to keep the communication honest while at the same time keeping the topic open for a future time, hopefully later in the interview.

Asking the child about his hobbies and interests serves at least two purposes. First, the clinician learns important information about the type and difficulty level of activities in which the child engages willingly and spontaneously. Children with motor coordination problems may shy away from physical games and sports. Children with delayed development may choose activities that are less demanding. In the same way, asking about a child's usual playmates can provide information about the extent to which a child is developing parallel to his age cohorts as well as offering some insight into his social development. A second benefit of inquiring after a child's hobbies and avocations is to give the clinician a chance to interact with the child when the topic is nonthreatening and is more likely to involve success experiences than failure experiences. Of course this information should always be corroborated by the parents. Children may be likely to use fantasy to cover perceived deficits. The clumsy child may report that he is a soccer star or the lonely child may report that she has many friends who come over to her house every day after school.

Further inquiries about social relationships can provide useful information. The number and age of friends has already been mentioned. The quality of these relationships should also be assessed. This can be done by asking the child what he does with his friends, how he compares himself to his friends, and what he likes or dislikes about various individuals in his social environment. Conflict resolution involves skills that require certain levels of cognitive skills. By age eight, the child should be able to resolve most minor disputes in games or sports without appealing to an adult, unless the other party is intransigent. By age 12 years, adult intervention in conflict resolution of minor disputes should be unnecessary. Consistent reliance on an adult in these matters should be assessed further to determine if the child is overly psychologically dependent on certain adults or cognitively unable to problem solve in these situations.

As part of the evaluation, the clinician can pose situations to the child and ask how he would resolve them. Very young children may answer with magical thinking. For example, when asked "What would you do if an older

The Interview and History

child takes away your toy?", the four-year-old replies, "I would turn into He-Man and make him give it back." Here it is less problematic than if a seven-year-old gave that reply. Young children between the ages of six and eight may reply that they would get their parents or older siblings to retrieve the toy. Children older than that may demonstrate a different form of thinking by replying that they might first try to reason with the offender or enlist the help of their friends before seeking adult help.

The clinician should inquire about functioning in several different areas. These areas include, but are not limited to the referral problem; the interests of the child; attitudes toward school and performance in school; peer relationships; sibling relationships; relationships with parents and other adult authorities; fears, worries, and concerns of the child; likes and dislikes about himself; the events that elicit emotional responses and the behaviors associated with those emotional responses; the presence of somatic concerns; the aspirations and goals of the child; and the presence and content of fantasy. In older children the areas of interest include heterosexual relationships, attitudes and concerns about sex, and drug and alcohol use.

Another important aspect of the interview is the setting. A professional office with respectable books, a desk, and diplomas on the wall is appropriate for the evaluation of adults and older adolescents. It may be inappropriate for the evaluation of younger children. Some clinicians use a playroom for the evaluation of children. This type of setting can certainly help the child feel more at ease, but the clutter of a playroom may distract the child from the task at hand. If a room other than an office is used, there should be a minimum of distracting toys and artwork. If the office is used, the clinician should move out from behind the desk. A small table that allows the clinician and child to sit side by side may help lessen the professional distance. As much as possible, the clinician should be sitting on the same level as the child so as not to appear intimidating. It should be noted that there are instances when allowing younger children the opportunity to play with toys can offer valuable clinical information.

During the interview, the child may express a desire to tell a secret. Usually, but not always, this signals the communication of important information. The clinician wants information but she should not allow this desire to cause her to make promises that cannot be kept. Secrets involving physical or sexual abuse cannot be kept. Secrets that involve information pertinent to the diagnosis or treatment should not be kept. If the child brings up the topic of secrets, the clinician should inquire as to who the secret needs to exclude. This is followed by a brief discussion of how any secrets that involve harm to the child have to be told to someone. The clinician may respond that there are laws that may prevent keeping the secret totally. However, although she cannot promise that she will tell no one, she can promise that the child will play a role in deciding who needs to be told.

INTERVIEWING THE PARENTS

Interviewing the parents provides two important types of information regarding the child. First, the parents can provide the information necessary to conducting a clinical history. Second, the parents provide information regarding the current problem which the child may be unwilling or unable to provide. As an auxiliary notion, the behavior of the parents plays a large role in the determination of the behavior of the child. The parents comprise much of the social environment of child, especially younger children, and the behavior of the parents may be eliciting or maintaining problematic behaviors in the child.

When interviewing the parents, it is important to avoid the use of judgmental behavior, not only in regard to the parents' behavior and attitudes, but also in regard to the behavior of the child. The nonjudgmental stance of the clinician may be difficult to maintain in the face of parents who have already labelled their child's behavior as abnormal or who are demonstrating behavior at odds with the clinician's view of appropriate child-rearing practices. During the early stages of the evaluation, subtle cues from the clinician may cause the parent to color the information provided to the clinician. This situation is to be avoided. Treatment cannot begin until the assessment is concluded in an atmosphere of impartiality.

The notable exception to this general principle exists in the areas of child sexual or physical abuse. Child abuse occurs in every level of socioeconomic status (SES) and may be uncovered in every clinical setting. The clinician who assesses or treats children as part of her clinical practice should be knowledgeable about the local laws regarding reporting child abuse and neglect. The telephone number for the agency to which reports are made should be available in every clinic. It is the legal duty as well as the ethical and moral responsibility of clinicians to report and intervene in child abuse cases as soon as the degree of suspicions specified by local law is reached. Child abuse has profound emotional implications in our culture, and clinicians cannot expect to be immune from them. However, the clinician should desensitize herself to these issues to facilitate a professional approach and maintain impartiality.

These issues become especially important because the first signs of child abuse or neglect may be the symptoms for which a child is referred for evaluation. Proper nutrition is essential to the normal neurobehavioral development of the child, and neglect can result in nutritionally based mental retardation. Physical abuse is a significant source of child head injury in this country, and a clinician who detects cognitive impairment secondary to suspected head injuries needs to evaluate carefully the etiology of those injuries. Sexual abuse can result in bizarre or age-inappropriate behavior. Again, it is usually the mental health clinician who first evaluates such a child.

INTERVIEWING SCHOOL PERSONNEL

School is another source of information in assessing the child. Obtaining information from the school can do much to help redress the imbalance inherent in relying solely on the parents as informants. The school can offer a substantial amount of information relevant to the proper diagnosis of the child, as it occupies a large part of a child's life that should not be ignored. The activities of school represent a significant sample of a child's behavior under varying conditions. At school, there are opportunities to evaluate the child's social and academic behavior as well as the more general aspects of cognitive functioning.

Unfortunately, school personnel and health professionals historically do not have a good relationship. Often the school personnel mistrust the health professionals and may feel that the professionals are condescending to them or that health professionals blame them for causing or not adequately managing the child's behavior. School personnel may also feel that health professionals do not understand the school situation and that they are likely to make unrealistic suggestions.

Because of these considerations, clinicians who assess and treat children need to be familiar with the local school settings. The best way to have a good relationship with a school is to develop the relationship over time. The clinician should demonstrate respect for the teacher's perspective and views, and remember that the teachers are the experts in the schools and that the health professionals are essentially outsiders. When the clinician leaves a meeting with school personnel, she may feel that she has given the best advice, but she should also remember that after she leaves, the school personnel must remain in the situation.

The school is most obviously useful in providing information regarding past and current grades and the scores on standardized academic achievement tests. However, the school personnel can also provide information derived from direct observation. It is useful to question school personnel about the usual activity level of the child and whether there have been any recent changes. The teacher can also be questioned as to the attentional capacity of the child and how easy or difficult it is to motivate the child. The teachers can offer information regarding the emotional adjustment of the child, including his tolerance for frustration, amount of impulsivity, and any disorders of mood. Teachers can also provide information regarding the social functioning of the child. For example, how well does the child relate to peers? Is his play characterized by excessive aggression? Is he usually a passive participant in play activities?

For older children, the clinician may not be able to identify a single teacher who can provide the needed information. The school counselor or homeroom teacher may be able to provide the information. The clinician can inquire into the child's participation in extracurricular activities. Not all children will possess the dexterity to be successful at sports, but any recent changes in the types or amount of extracurricular activity may be associated with psychiatric or neurological problems. The withdrawn, depressed child may discontinue his social and extracurricular activities. The child with developing neurological problems in motor activity or coordination may discontinue sports activities.

OBTAINING THE HISTORY

The history of the child begins with the history of the parents. Many neurological and psychiatric disorders have genetic components and a complete history of other family members with the same or similar problems should be obtained. It is important to obtain information regarding the parents' primary families as well as information regarding the parents' social and academic history. The parents' vocational and avocational interests should be assessed. Although the child operates in the same macroculture that we all do, he also operates in the subculture that is unique to his family. Reports of poor performance in school are evaluated differently when the child is raised in a family where both parents possess postsecondary education and in which education is valued than when the child is raised in a family where the parents did not finish school and do not place a value on education.

The clinician should obtain a review of the medical history of the parents and a review of the psychological problems that may have been experienced by the parents. Again, congruence of the child's presenting problems with those of the parents may suggest a genetic etiology. Incongruence may be a sign either of the environmental influence on the problem or of an acquired organic etiological influence.

The parents' main concerns about the child can be elicited in an interview format or through the use of a structured questionnaire such as the Personality Inventory for Child (Wirt, Lachar, Klinedinst, & Seat, 1984) or the Achenbach Child Behavior Checklist (Achenbach & Edelbrock, 1983). We recommend the use of both types of assessment. The questionnaires can

The Interview and History

help survey many different areas of problem behaviors, but the interviews will allow the clinician to evaluate the problems in more depth and with greater specificity.

The history of the development of the presenting problem can be very helpful in determining the diagnosis. The clinician should inquire as to the first time that the problem behavior appeared and whether the onset was acute or insidious. It is not necessarily true that problems that develop acutely always have an organic etiology and that problems that develop in an insidious fashion always have an environmental etiology. For example, although a head injury resulting from an automobile accident is an acute event, the adjustment problems exhibited by the mildly head-injured child may develop over time as difficulties in learning new material at school arise or as the cognitive and perceptual demands of interpersonal functioning cause increasing frustration in the child. In a similar manner, although epileptic seizures may first occur for purely organic reasons, the response of the environment to the seizures may increase or decrease the frequency with which future seizures occur, or the initiation of a seizure episode may become conditioned to a particular set of environmental variables such as family arguments or the threat of a stressful situation.

The overall purpose of the history is to obtain information relevant to the diagnosis of the patient and to the decision to refer to a neurologist or neuropsychologist for a more specialized evaluation. The history taken from the parents usually provides information in response to the questions. The history taken from the child also allows the clinician an opportunity to evaluate aspects of motor behavior and language skill and other associated behaviors. Although the patient, especially an adolescent, may be able to provide a reliable history, it is always wise to obtain an ancillary history from the parents.

Current Complaints

As mentioned previously, the first part of a history involves a specification of the current complaints and the history of the development of those complaints. By interviewing both the parents and the child, the clinician can determine who "owns" the problem. Does the child recognize a problem? Do the parents? Is the patient court-referred or did the school recognize the problem and suggest the evaluation to the parents? Can the informants relate the problem behavior to an etiological event? Here it is important for the clinician to probe for a history of events such as mild head injury or exposure to solvents which the informants may not associate with behavior problems.

The clinician should also determine the environmental and behavioral concomitants of the problem. Does the problem seem to occur more frequently under certain conditions than under others? What are the responses of others to the problem being exhibited? Have there been previous attempts to treat the problem? What was the effect of the treatment? Behavioral problems that are resistant to psychologically based treatments may be due to organic variables, although it is certainly true that lack of response to treatment may also signal an incorrect or inadequately implemented treatment.

Family History

The family history can be extremely important in the evaluation of the patient. Many psychiatric disorders, such as bipolar affective disorder, and many neurological disorders, such as epilepsy, are either known or are thought to be have genetic components. Knowledge of the presence or absence of these disorders in either the immediate or extended family can be helpful in diagnosing or ruling out such a disorder. Obtaining a history of the immediate family, especially of the siblings, will also provide information regarding the family social structure. To whom does the child relate best? Is the child differentially obedient when with siblings or peers versus when alone? Do the siblings have any similar problems?

Prenatal History

The mother is usually the best informant in this area, but even here she may not be totally reliable. It is useful for the clinician to encourage the mother to check any details of which she may not be sure, as well as details of which she is relatively certain. The mother may have copies of the prenatal record which will document the events in the current chronology. The clinician should also inquire as to whether the mother worked during pregnancy and if her occupation exposed her to industrial solvents, toxins, or other chemicals. Whether or not the mother was outside the country during the pregnancy is important, especially if she was in an undeveloped country in which she may have been exposed to infectious diseases.

The use of drugs by the mother should also be determined. This includes prescription, over-the-counter, and recreational drugs. Fetal alcohol syndrome is an extreme example of the significant cognitive effects of the mother's behavior on the child's later behavior, but lesser amounts of alcohol may be associated with more subtle signs of cognitive dysfunction. Mothers who smoke cigarettes run the risk of producing children with lower body weight and cognitive difficulties.

Because of the relationship between the cognitive and body weight effects of maternal prenatal behavior, the clinician should also inquire as to the body weight at birth. Initial denials of prenatal alcohol use may turn to admissions that she had only two or three drinks a day during pregnancy. Complications in pregnancy or in the birth process itself may result in later cognitive difficulties. Was the gestational age young, normal, or late? Were there any complications resulting from the use of an anesthetic during delivery? Was the use of forceps required?

Early History

Depending on the age of the child, the early history may turn out to be the complete history. However, regardless of the present age of the child, the early history needs to be delineated. There is some variability in the age at which developmental milestones are met, but significant delays may signal the presence of a neurological disorder or may predict the later occurrence of neuropsychological difficulties.

The optimal situation is one in which the child is seen in a clinic where his development has been followed over time and where there are records documenting early developmental history. Unfortunately, this is rarely the case. A desirable situation is one in which the accompanying parent brings along copies of the developmental history of the child. These records, taken contemporaneously with development, are more reliable than retrospective reports. Although retrospective reports are the norm, they are less desirable because the recent events involving abnormal behavior or poor academic functioning may influence the shape and content of the reports.

Be that as it may, if records are unavailable, the clinician should inquire as to the developmental milestones and the ages at which these were reached. It is insufficient merely to ask if the milestones were met at the usual time. Generally, a parent's sense of "the usual time" is generated from a comparison with siblings or from informal comparisons with neighbors' children. Comparison among siblings of the age at which milestones were met can be useful in determining whether the child's development varies from "normal" as a function of genetic factors or as a function of something unique to the child who is the identified patient. But these data should still be compared to normative values to help determine whether any delays occurred.

The clinician should ask at what age the child sat up unassisted, first walked, and first talked. Although many parents may not be able to provide specificity, the clinician should inquire as to the quality of developmental speech, for example, when the child paired words together and spoke in sentences. The quality of the child's posture and gait should be determined. The presence of early developmental anomalies may mean that there is a neurological substrate to the child's complaints and therefore increases the probability that referral to a neurologist or neuropsychologist should be made.

If the child is younger, the use of a developmental schedule such as the Alpern–Boll (Alpern & Shearer, 1980) may be useful. The Alpern–Boll is an attempt to systematically obtain information regarding the developmental age of a child. It is meant to inventory various skills of children from birth to the age of nine years. It takes between 20 to 40 minutes to administer. Rather than provide a single number to describe the developmental age of the child, the Alpern–Boll provides age equivalencies for five areas of development: Physical, Self-Help, Social, Academic, and Communication. The Alpern–Boll also provides an IQ equivalency score; however, this score should not be interpreted strictly. Whenever possible the IQ of the child should be determined by a formal test of intellectual functioning.

By separating the assessment of the development of the child into five areas, a greater range of information is obtained. Many children will not develop consistently across all areas. The Alpern–Boll will allow the clinician to determine if there is a serious discrepancy among the areas of development. The test can be administered by interviewing the child's primary caregiver, or more preferably, by direct observation of the child in situations evaluated by the test.

Each area of the Alpern–Boll is divided into levels or stages. The administration is terminated when a child fails all items at two consecutive age levels. Each section has between 34 and 39 items, and there are about three items for each age level. The age levels increase by six-month intervals. Because there are only three items for every six months, interpretation of the Alpern–Boll should be conducted cautiously in the context of a more complete evaluation of other areas of the child's functioning.

Reversal in development should be viewed as a red flag by the clinician. Some variability in the age at which children meet developmental milestones may be due to familial (genetic) factors; some might be due to environmental factors. For example, the siblings of a child patient may have exhibited the same three-month delay in exhibiting speech without showing the later academic difficulties shown by the patient. Or as another example, a child who is raised in a family where both parents work during the day and the caretaker is a nearly deaf grandparent may show delays in language acquisition as the result of environmental factors.

Just as all children do not reach miletones at the same age, a single child may not reach all classes of milestones at the prescribed time. Many different factors impinge on development, and a child may show early development in one area, normal development in another area, and tardy development in a third area. The age at which a child first sits, walks, and performs other aspects of gross motor development is less important than the age at which she learns to use her hands. The most important two areas are the extent to which a child is responsive to her environment and can maintain concentration on a single task.

If there are siblings for a child who reportedly met milestones late, or if data are available on the parent's milestones, patterns of familial tardiness would be less cause for concern. Prematurely born children also tend to be somewhat late in reaching milestones. The milestones are better thought of as occurring at a certain age past conception rather than past birth. As a general rule of thumb, one can subtract the amount of time that the child was premature in making judgments of tardiness.

Early development is largely assessed as a function of the child's response to environmental stimulation. Many of these aspects may not be noticed or recorded by parents, and for these reasons, the history may be difficult to determine. However, if the child was followed at a healthy baby clinic or if the parents have kept a baby book, the clinician can ask to see the medical records or the baby book and assess the milestones. Unfortunately, the baby book is more likely to be kept for the first child than for subsequent offspring. This is a corollary of the well-known observation that baby pictures exist in abundance and decrease in number for each younger sibling, so that pictures of the fourth child may consist of a birth picture and yearly school portraits.

The clinician should also inquire as to early personal and interpersonal development. If the child is of school age, were there signs of school phobia or greater than usual separation anxiety? Was the child able to form friendships? What was the quality of these relationships, and more importantly, has the quality deteriorated recently? Is the child irritable? Here, questionnaires such as the Achenbach Child Behavior Checklist or the Personality Inventory for Children can be very useful in comparing the current level of personal and interpersonal development of the child to normative data.

Academic History

For children who are old enough to be in school (which is at a younger and younger age as daycare and preschool centers proliferate), it is necessary to obtain an academic history. The clinician should pay attention both to the summary grades obtained and the narratives provided by teachers. When possible, data should also be obtained from the results of standardized testing. Grades assigned by teachers vary greatly among teachers and may even vary among different children with the same teacher as attempts are made to reward effort rather than achievement. For those reasons, objective data in the form of standardized test scores are desirable.

The school personnel can be useful in the assessment of the child. Although most teachers and school counselors are not trained to observe and record behaviors associated with organic problems in children, they tend to be accurate judges of what is abnormal behavior in a child. Teachers observe groups of children in cohorts. They are aware of the normal variability present in child behavior and development and can usually discriminate abnormal behavior from variants of normal behavior.

Teachers have a greater knowledge of normal behavior than do many parents, who have only their own children as a reference. Teachers are also likely to be aware of the latest trends and fads. Grammar school children, no less than high school adolescents, have their own behavioral norms, including those for dress and relationships with adults. The clinician usually becomes aware of these norms a little behind the school teacher. What may at first seem deviant to a clinician may after consultation with the child's teacher turn out to be an outlier in normal trends.

Information from the school represents data gathered from a large behavioral and contextual sample. The behavior of a child in a clinical evaluation is the behavior of the child in a one-to-one setting with all of the intimidating surroundings of the hospital, mental health center, or private practice office. With the possible exception of psychotic children, the importance for the future of the child of an evaluation by a mental health professional does not usually escape even the most disobedient, hyperactive, or disordered child. His behavior during the evaluation is likely to reflect this fact.

Clinicians can partially overcome this tendency to meet social and contextual expectations by spending increasing amounts of time with the child. In essence, the longer evaluation wears down the child's wariness; unfortunately, the clinician's resolve and motivation may also be worn down. Another method of overcoming the contingencies for exhibiting behavior in accord with social desirability is to gather information from various sources, while paying careful attention to the contextual variables and stimulus characteristics of the information sources. In that way, the clinician can begin to understand the functional relationships between the child's behavior and the contingencies eliciting and maintaining the behavior.

Occupational History

Obtaining an occupational history in a child is not as ludicrous as it may seem. However, the clinician needs to broaden his concept of what constitutes an occupation. Younger children have as their occupation the completion of chores. The clinician can inquire as to the responsibilities of the child in the home. Here, it is important to consider the degree of responsibility given the child and the child's response to that responsibility. Can the child perform chores independently or must supervision be provided? Can the child remember the instructions from occasion to occasion or must reminders be given? Can the child be trusted to care for a pet? Equally important is whether there have been any recent changes in these variables.

Older children may have paper routes, baby-sitting services, or lawn care operations. Again, it is important to evaluate the ability of the child to perform these chores independently and to determine the presence of any changes. Can the child handle her personal finances? Can she take responsibility for her clothing and personal hygiene? Is the child able to problem-solve in work situations in an age-appropriate fashion?

Sexual History

If clinicians are sometimes squeamish about taking an adequate sexual history in adults, they completely avoid taking a sexual history in children. In our culture, children are thought to be free from the "corrupting" influences of sexual behavior. In fact, any exhibition of sexual behavior by children may cause parents to bring a child in for evaluation. However, parents may also be reluctant to describe their child's sexual behavior to a health authority, and it may be necessary for the clinician to breach the silence. Curiosity and verbal inquiries about sexual matters are normal and are not a cause for concern in most cases. Actually engaging in sexual behavior, especially if that behavior continues after parental admonishments, is problematic and may be a reflection of clandestine sexual interactions with adults or of organic etiologies. Treating the assessment of sexual behavior in a matter-of-fact tone can help induce parents to provide the necessary information and provide a nonjudgmental atmosphere for the child to relate the sexual history.

In our society adolescents may become sexually active before the prevailing cultural norms allow such behavior. The clinician can begin inquiries into sexual behavior by first inquiring about the dating and heterosexual-social behavior of the child. The extent to which child client–clinician interactions are confidential vary from state to state, and the clinician should be knowledgeable about the statutory limitations on confidentiality. This information should be given to the child before the evaluation begins. The child exhibits changes in sexual behavior as the result of normal maturation. However, abrupt changes or changes inconsistent with societal values should be carefully evaluated. Hypersexuality may be the result of bipolar affective disorder–mania or of subcortical dysfunction.

Medical History

Many states require physical examinations of children at specified transitions in the educational system. As a result, children may have had a more recent physical examination than most adults. It should be pointed out that many of these physical examinations are cursory or may have a focus outside the detection of neurological abnormalities. If the mental health clinician suspects an organic etiology for the identified psychological problems, referral to a qualified pediatric specialist is in order.

Taking an adequate medical history of the child includes examination of previous medical records. Some infectious diseases may have central nervous system effects that do not become evident until later in the developmental sequence. For example, early childhood measles or sustained high fevers may show effects when the child fails to keep pace with her cohorts in academic achievement. The use of medication, both prescription and nonprescription, should also be assessed. The relationship of the presenting problem to the medication should be determined.

Current Situation

Finally, the current situation of the child should be assessed. The number and relationship of people with whom the child lives should be documented. The presence and level of stress in the home environment can be an important etiological factor in the development of any behavioral or emotional symptoms. Children are more sensitive to the problems of other individuals and may show signs of stress before the adults do. Legal difficulties of the child and of the other people living with the child should be determined. It is a fact of our current society that many children live with single parents or with combined or blended families. The extent to which a child has adapted to new living situations, including new stepparents, has a large influence on the emergence of abnormal behavior.

Suggested Structured Interview

Appendix A contains a suggested structure for the interview of the parents. In this structured interview, there are questions to elicit information regarding many of the concerns discussed in the current chapter. There are also sections to allow recording some of the behavioral observations we feel are important. The individual clinician may want to revise the questionnaire to delete items that do not pertain to the population usually served in her practice. Alternately, the clinician may want to add items that are not thought to be sufficiently covered in the suggested format. This particular interview format is suggested only as a starting point, and revisions are recommended.

CONCLUSIONS

The history can be an important part of evaluating a child, for multiple reasons. The most obvious is that the DSM III-R diagnostic system is based on history as much as it is based on current clinical presentation. It is by knowing the history that we can place the current condition of the child into context and thereby obtain a greater understanding of the child. It is not enough to know that a child is presenting with difficulty in the ability to carry digits across unit places in mathematical operations. We also need to know if the child was slow to develop verbal skills or demonstrated difficulty with visual-spatial tasks such as puzzles. We can then begin to generate hypotheses that can be evaluated during the extended mental status exam.

The history serves to alert the clinician to problematic areas in the child's profile of skills and difficulties. The information derived from the history can be considered only anecdotal. But it is useful in planning whether to investigate in greater depth certain areas covered in the mental status exam. In a similar fashion, the history can be used to help streamline the mental status exam. If a child has a history of good verbal expressive skills and if there are no reported changes in skill level, that aspect of the mental status exam can be shortened somewhat. One should never use information from the history to support a decision to delete entirely a portion of the mental status exam. The history is verbal behavior and, as such, has all of the associated problems of reliability and accuracy. Clinicians who ignore the history will conduct redundant mental status exams or, worse, incomplete mental status exams.

7
The Mental Status Exam in Children

The mental status exam is the means by which the clinician attempts to evaluate the cognitive, emotional, and behavioral condition of the patient by employing a series of semisystematic methods of assessment. Most of the procedures in a mental status exam are informal, but are meant to provide coherence, structure, and fullness to the understanding of the patient's clinical condition. As such the mental status exam often includes some short standardized procedures as well as short tests with normative data for interpretive purposes.

There are as many different forms of the mental status exam as there are clinicians. However, the better mental status exams offer a fairly complete sample of relevant areas and are geared toward the developmental, intellectual, and emotional condition of the patient. For many mental status exams, interpretation is by reference to a set of informal, internal norms that are gathered by the clinician as the result of training experiences and later professional activity. The clinician comes to associate certain performances with impairment, or in some cases, with particular diagnoses.

Children have greater variability than do adults in cognitive, behavioral, and emotional functioning. On the one hand, this fact may seem to argue in favor of greater use of standardized procedures in assessing children. Standardized procedures have the benefit of allowing comparisons of the individual to a larger number of patients than might otherwise be possible by a single clinician. However, the interpretation of norms has at its base the idea of an averaged performance with the attendant problems of masking individual variability. So although the increased variability of children makes the use of standardized procedures more important, it also has the effect of making it more important for the clinician to be open to individual differences that may not have diagnostic significance. Stated another way, statistics describing variability (standard deviation, error of measurement) are as important as statistics describing central tendency (mean, mode).

As well as having an armamentarium of standardized procedures, the clinician who evaluates or treats children should have a fair understanding of normal child development. There is no easy way to acquire this understanding. However, it begins with a familiarity with current developmental theories, whether this familiarity was gained through formal didactic training or through self-study and reading. Regardless of where the child clinician begins the study of developmental processes, the study is not ever complete as each of the clinician's new experiences with children in clinical settings should be integrated into this knowledge. Just as researchers in developmental theory are never satisfied with a current theory, so should clinicians continually revise their internal norms on the basis of changes in the literature and on the basis of experience.

There has always been tension between proponents of objective standardized assessment and proponents of clinical, intuitive qualitative assessment. Although it is not the purpose of this volume to resolve or even to adequately address the issue, it is important for a clinician to require that clinical hunches and "intuition" be subjected to the same sort of public examination by which objective assessment methods are evaluated. That is, clinical, informal assessment methods should be capable of verbal description and repetition. If a clinician includes among her assessment methods a game of catch with the child, the means of evaluating the performance of the child during the ballgame should be explicitly stated, such as whether the child throws or catches the ball consistently with the same hand and whether he can form graceful, integrated motor activities into a successful chain.

As with the adult form, the child mental status exam is best conceptualized as a hierarchical set of procedures that systematically evaluates the relevant areas of mental functioning through the use of standardized assessment methods and more informal procedures. The child mental status exam should be tailored to the child's age, to the level of cooperation elicited from the child, and to the emotional status of the child. Simpler, more molecular aspects of mental functioning are evaluated first, and depending on the outcome of these evaluations, more complex, molar aspects are evaluated later. Although some knowledge of the presenting problem can help focus the evaluation, the clinician should maintain a flexible attitude toward uncovering both strengths and weaknesses.

Several types of children should be considered for an extended mental status exam.

1. Any child with a history of a central nervous system disorder should receive an extended mental status exam as part of the initial evaluation. The central nervous system disorder can be in the form of a developmental disorder such as mental retardation or in the form of an acquired lesion such as that resulting from a head injury or cerebral tumor.

2. Any child with a history of a CVA (cerebral vascular accident) should receive an extended mental status exam. Although CVAs or stroke are much more common in middle-aged adults than in children, they can occur.

3. Children with a suspected central nervous system disorder should also receive an extended mental status exam. Suspicion of a central nervous system disorder can come from reports of dizziness, unexplained nausea, headaches, or periods of inattention. Reports of untreated mild head injury will also signify the need for an extended mental status exam. Furthermore some medical disorders such as poorly controlled diabetes or meningitis are an indication of the need to perform an extended mental status exam.

4. An extended mental status exam should also be performed when the parents or teachers report sudden changes in emotional status, in behavior patterns, in school performance, or in everyday aspects of cognitive functioning such as memory. Organic etiologies are not the only reason why these symptoms may occur, and a good functional analysis will help delineate the environmental factors related to the changes.

5. Reports of recent changes in sensory function should be followed by an extended mental status exam.

6. Finally, reports of psychiatric symptoms will need further evaluation including an extended mental status exam.

There are many differences between children and adults, but one thing they share is the tendency for organic problems to present first with abnormal behavior that may be confused with a strictly psychiatric diagnosis.

ESSENTIALS OF THE EXTENDED MENTAL STATUS EXAM FOR CHILDREN

There appear to be relationships between certain sets of gross behavioral symptoms and certain types of cognitive disorders. However, these relationships do not tend to exist in a one-to-one correspondence. Multiple disorders may have similar behavioral symptoms with only a few distinct differences to separate them. On the other hand, not all individuals with the same cognitive disorders will show the same gross behavioral symptoms. Therefore, it is wise for the child clinician to approach each mental status exam with an open mind. Information from the history or the referral source may help focus the evaluation, but the information should not serve as a set of blinders, limiting what the clinician is assessing.

The mental status exam is actually a systematic method for organizing one's thoughts, observations, and procedures. The optimal mental status exam is organized analogously to our theories of brain/behavior relationships, namely in an hierarchical system. Beginning at the simplest levels and working up through more complex levels can simplify the evaluation. For example, if the child is unable to write letters from dictation, there is no need to assess the ability to write sentences from dictation. Working in this fashion will also allow the clinician to differentiate the reason for failure on a more complex item. If the child was able to repeat words but unable to repeat a short paragraph, the deficit may be in memory span rather than in auditory discrimination and comprehension.

The first step in an mental status exam is to assess the level of consciousness. However, it is unlikely that a general child clinician seeing children in an outpatient setting will be asked to evaluate a child with a disturbance of consciousness. For that reason and because procedures for the evaluation of level of consciousness are discussed elsewhere (Berg, Franzen, & Wedding, 1987), those procedures will not be discussed here.

It may also be useful to assess orientation in older children. The clinician can inquire as to the date, time, and place of the evaluation. Most children should be able to give their name. Older children should be able to give the name of the place where the evaluation is taking place.

ATTENTION

Attention is the first aspect of cognitive functioning likely to be assessed in an outpatient setting. Part of the assessment of attention is based on qualitative observations by the clinician. The clinician will want to note the relative ease or difficulty with which she is able to gain the attention of the child. The assessment of whether or not the child can follow the examiner's verbal communication is tempered by the later evaluation of receptive speech functions. Children may be more easily distracted than adults, so it is more important that the office be relatively free of distracting stimuli. A relatively quiet room with a thick door that does not allow sounds from the hallway to enter is desirable.

Can the child be oriented to the task by simply calling his name? If not, how much stimulation is required to obtain the child's attention? Temporal aspects of attention are also important. How long can the child appear to concentrate on a single task? Does the child need to be reoriented each time the procedure changes slightly? Furthermore, the clinician will want to note how long the child can maintain attention before it starts to wane. By making subtle notes on the evaluation protocol, the clinician can document the time periods during which attention is maintained. Another consideration is the extent to which fatigue interferes with attention and at what time fatigue sets in. If the child is distracted by noises in the hall, how difficult is it to return to task? What procedures were needed to redirect the child?

Standardized procedures for the assessment of attention include the Digit Span subtest from the Wechsler Intelligence Scale for Children-Revised (WISC-R). The scoring procedures from the WISC-R can be borrowed for the purposes of interpretation. *If the clinician intends later to use the WISC-R as part of the evaluation, she would be wise to prepare a parallel form for the purposes of evaluating attention here.*

The ability to sustain attention is sometimes called vigilance. Usually the period of evaluation here is no longer than 30 seconds. Although vigilance is best evaluated in a laboratory with special equipment, the clinician can use some behavioral procedures for a rough evaluation of vigilance aspects of attention. For example, the Random Letters Procedure can be used. In the Random Letters Procedure the clinician has prepared a list of about 75 letters in which a target letter (e.g., the letter "F") appears about 15 times. The clinician then reads the letters out to the child, asking him to tap on the table every time the letter F is spoken. To perform a finer discrimination of vigilance, the clinician can also have letters that appear 10 or 15 times during the series and ask the child to tap when those letters are spoken. It may be that making the event less frequent greatly disrupts vigilance.

If the child is old enough to be able to perform subtraction, attention can be assessed by using a serial subtraction task. Have the child start at 30 and subtract 2 each time. Or as a more complex form of the task, have the child start at 50 and subtract 3. Remember the age of the child and the language that is used to describe subtraction to children. The instructions may read something like, "I'd like you to do an arithmetic puzzle. Please start at 30 and take away 2, what do you have? Now take away 2 from that, what do you have? Good. Now keep taking away 2 each time and tell what the new number is." For adolescents, the clinician can have the patient start at 100 and subtract 7. This procedure requires several skills including arithmetic, memory, and mental control. Impaired performance may not be due solely to deficits in attention. However, by comparing the results of this procedure to the results of other aspects of the mental status exam, the possibility of an attentional deficit can be surmised.

LANGUAGE

Because language skills are required during the entire mental status exam, evaluation of language skills is not confined to this particular section but

The Mental Status Exam in Children 75

instead take place whenever the child is asked to use his receptive or expressive language skills. Be that as it may, the procedures described here can help systematize the evaluation of language skills.

Generally speaking, language skills can be divided into receptive and expressive areas. Receptive language skills and the ability to perceive and understand language include both spoken and written verbal information. Of course in younger children, the evaluation of receptive language skills will be confined to spoken information. In an analogous manner, expressive language skills contain both written and spoken communication, although again for younger children only their ability to speak is assessed. Consistent with the overall scheme for the mental status exam, the assessment of language begins at the simplest level and proceeds to more complex levels. Prior to the evaluation, the clinician can prepare cards that contain appropriate stimuli for the evaluation. The present text gives some examples of stimuli that can be adapted to the needs of the clinician.

To assess auditory discrimination, the clinician can ask the patient to repeat a brief series of phonemes—"A, F, M, O, R". The clinician can then ask the child (if he is old enough) to read those letters from a card. By comparing performance on the two tasks, it may be possible to begin differentiation between receptive and expressive language skills. Next the clinician can repeat the same procedure using words—"ball, fun, apple."

To assess more complex comprehension, the clinician can give the patient a series of verbal commands progressing from simple to more complex. An example of a useful sequence is:

1. Please stand up.
2. Give me the pencil.
3. Fold the piece of paper in half and give it to me.
4. If today is Friday, raise both arms; otherwise raise only one arm.
5. Put your right hand on your left shoulder.

Notice that the early statements required single direct requests, and that later statements, although requiring simple motor responses, were based on the understanding of conditional statements, the use of information external to the evaluation setting, and the understanding of spatial relationships.

In assessing expressive speech the clinician can ask the patient to name some simple objects from photographs or line drawings. Here the visual system must be intact for adequate performance, and the results should be interpreted in that light. These pictures can be mounted on 3 × 5 cards. Using the same set of cards for different clients can give the clinician some local norms.

In assessing receptive and expressive speech, a repetition task can be very useful. Starting with simple words, moving through more difficult words to simple phrases and then to sentences, the clinician can assess where in the scheme of complexity the performance of the child breaks down. The following sequence given first orally and then in a written form can be useful:

1. The yellow ball.
2. Sugar and spice.
3. Yes, I do.
4. The girl hit a homerun.
5. All dogs chase cats.
6. The robin built a nest for its baby.

In evaluating the child's speech output, the clinician should pay attention to pronunciation as well as to aspects of speech regulation. The ability of the child to produce meaningful speech by modulating tone of voice and rhythm yields important information. Elements to look for include abrupt changes in tone or rhythm, lack of rhythm variability, lack of intonation to signal the end of a sentence or to convey meaning accurately, and monotone productions. Note separately whether the use of tonal and rhythmic aspects of speech to convey meaning is absent or whether the meaning conveyed by rhythm and tone is inaccurate or inappropriate. The two sets of conditions may have different interpretations. The lack of tonal and rhythmic modulation may be related to a right hemisphere lesion, but the inappropriate modulation may be due to a frontal lesion.

The more functional aspects of speech can be evaluated by asking the child to describe the contents of a picture that contains more than one activity. These pictures can be found in popular magazines and mounted on index cards. The clinician can also assess spontaneous speech skills by asking the child to describe his room at home or a favorite television program. Here the clinician should be evaluating multiple aspects of speech production. Some pertinent aspects include the ability to string words together into meaningful units, the ability to match appropriately the tone of voice to the content of the speech, and the ability to speak in a smooth manner. The latency between the command and the initiation of speech should be recorded. Finally, the clinician should note the relative richness or paucity of speech production.

The writing ability of the child can be assessed by following a procedure similar to the one described for spoken output. The child can be asked to write a series of letters, words, phrases, and sentences both from dictation and by copying the stimuli from a card. The child's behavioral product of written information is evaluated for length of time required for the child to write each item, the accuracy of output (spelling), and the presence of motor writing errors such as tremor or illegibility. For children older than eight or nine years, the clinician can ask for cursive writing as well as for printed responses.

MEMORY

Memory complaints are probably only slightly less common in children than in adults. Memory is not a unitary construct, and the assessment of memory should reflect this fact. If there are any concerns about memory, an evaluation using the instruments described in the chapter on memory assessment should be used. For the purposes of the mental status exam, memory assessment can be nonstandardized, although it should be structured. The different types of memory to be assessed include short-term memory and long-term memory. In addition, memory can be assessed in the verbal-auditory modality and the visual modality. Visual memory can be assessed for designs, colors, or spatial relationships. Finally, delayed memory following a period of interference can be assessed.

Repetition tasks can help assess short-term memory. The clinician can use a digit repetition procedure similar to the Digit Span although it should be noted that this type of assessment confounds memory with attention. Another task is to prepare a list of four unrelated words, such as "tree, book, happy, cookie." State the word list to the patient and ask him to repeat it. The patient can be asked to repeat the word list again after five minutes during which time interference is provided by continuing with the evaluation. Older children should be able to restate three of the four words after the five-minute delay. Younger children may be able to restate only two of the words.

Sometimes children who show impairment in their ability to remember a list of unrelated words will be able to remember more words if these are embedded in a meaningful context such as a short story. Therefore, even if the patient fails the word list procedure, he should be administered the short story procedure. In this procedure, a short story of no more than six sentences is read to the patient and the patient is asked to recall as much of it as possible. It is preferable to type the story on an index card to ensure that the clinician's verbalizations include all of the relevant information and to later check the response of the patient for detail.

Another type of memory is associative memory. To assess this type of memory, the clinician can type a list of five pairs of related and unrelated words. Using a mix of related (e.g., spoon–fork) and unrelated (e.g., tree–sign) words can help assess whether meaning facilitates associative memory for the child. Both words are given at first. Then only the first word is given and the child is asked to produce the second word. By repeating this procedure four or five times with the same list, an approximation of a learning curve can be derived.

Visual memory can be assessed partly by mounting three pictures from a magazine on cardboard. Then mount the three pictures on another piece of cardboard along with three distractors. Show the first set of pictures to the patient for 10 seconds. Then show the second set of pictures and ask the patient to identify the original pictures. A delayed procedure similar to that used in the assessment of verbal memory can be employed here. The clinician shows the second set of pictures again after five minutes and asks the child to pick out the original pictures. If the clinician attempts to compare the verbal delayed memory results with the visual delayed memory results, she needs to remember that the verbal task is recall memory and the visual task as described is recognition memory which should be more accurate than recall memory.

Visual memory can also be assessed by showing the patient an abstract design such as found in the Wechsler Memory Scale or Benton Visual Retention test. Then, after removing the design, ask the patient to draw it. Here memory is confounded with constructional abilities and interpretation of the child's performance should reflect that fact.

CONSTRUCTIONAL ABILITIES

Constructional abilities refer to the ability to draw or build two- or three-dimensional objects. Constructional abilities undergo much change during normal development, and assessment of constructional skills should be conducted with this fact in mind. Constructional abilities require an extensive complex of cortico-behavioral skills, and dysfunction in any one of the component skills can result in an impaired performance on constructional tasks. For that reason, many of the older screening tests relied exclusively on constructional tasks. We do not recommend such a simplistic approach but do recognize the strength of using constructional tasks in a mental status exam. The clinician should not interpret an impaired performance as evidence of right hemisphere dysfunction but should instead report the results simply as a behavioral deficit.

Drawing to command is an important aspect of assessing constructional skills. The clinician can ask the child to draw a horizontal line, a vertical line, a stick cross, a circle, a square, and a triangle. Older children can also be asked to draw a diamond and a stick man. Drawing from a stimulus can then be assessed using the same objects; this time the objects have been pre-drawn on an index card.

By age 2 the child should be able to copy a vertical line and a circle. By

$2\frac{1}{2}$ years of age, the child should be able to copy both a vertical and a horizontal line and to combine these into a cross. By age 3 years, the child should be able to draw an approximate square and a simple but recognizable stick man. Still older children can be expected to copy a simple abstract figure. Adolescents can be expected to copy a Greek cross.

Three-dimensional construction can be assessed by asking the child to copy block designs. At age 2 years, the child should be able to copy a "train" made of three blocks. By age 3 years, the train can be extended to five blocks. By age 4 years, the child should also be able to place a single block "smokestack" on the train.

HIGHER COGNITIVE FUNCTIONS

The assessment of higher cognitive functions is simplified by the developmentally normal absence of many of these functions in many children. However, for children older than 6 years of age, questions similar to those used in the Similarities subtest of the WISC-R can be used. Examples include, "How are spring and summer alike?" or, "How are a radio and a phonograph alike?" Simple verbal arithmetic questions can also be posed. For example, the clinician can ask, "What is 2 plus 4?", "How much is 7 take away 3?", or "If I give you one apple and your dad gives you two apples, how many apples do you have?". Again, it is a good idea for the clinician to have prepared a set of questions prior to the evaluation.

SUMMARY

The mental status exam for children is best conducted in a hierarchical fashion and is best interpreted in light of developmental considerations. The clinician should be cognizant of developmental norms when planning a mental status exam. At each stage of the exam, failure to perform adequately has implications for the following procedures. Interpretation should be kept to a minimum, and the report should describe the behavioral tasks attempted and the success or failure of the child on the item, rather naming the deficient neuropsychological skill or localizing the "lesion" responsible for the deficient performance.

8
The Wechsler Intelligence Scale for Children—Revised as a Screening Device

The Wechsler intelligence scales are frequently used as the core portion or cornerstone of a large number of complete neuropsychological evaluations. They have been found to provide a standardized series of tasks that can be used to evaluate the cognitive verbal and nonverbal skills as well as visual-motor skills of both children and adults. The Wechsler scales are generally seen to be sensitive to brain damage, since brain damage at any age can impair the ability to learn, to solve unfamiliar problems, and to think abstractly. The Wechsler Intelligence Scale for Children-Revised (WISC-R) (Wechsler, 1974) assesses these abilities and others quite well (Sattler, 1982).

The WISC-R was published 25 years after the publication of the Wechsler Intelligence Scale for Children (WISC) (Wechsler, 1949). The original WISC was published as a downward extension of an adult intelligence test, the Wechsler Bellevue Intelligence Scale. To simplify and make the adult test more appropriate for younger individuals, easier items were added to the low end of each of the subtests.

As a general rule, brain-injured children tend to show a good deal of variability in their WISC-R *subtest* scores. WISC-R IQ scores for children with brain injury may also show much variability, in some cases as much as 30 or more points. However, it is important to note that, in several instances, *there may be little if any difference between the WISC-R Verbal and Performance IQ scores.* Subtest scores may range from considerably above average to well below average. Even when brain-injured children perform in the average range, they may show specific difficulties such as deficits in attention and concentration. An overall reduction in the level of intelligence may be a key finding in some cases of brain damage.

Intelligence tests, such as the WISC-R, allow the clinician to assess not only patterns of test performance but also a number of qualitative indices that can reveal difficulties with cognitive efficiency and control (Sattler, 1982). Such observational indices include perseveration, confusion, conceptual and reasoning difficulties, and visual-motor difficulties. Some of these difficulties may reflect compensatory adjustments associated with brain injury whereas others can be a more direct expression of the damage.

WISC-R VERBAL-PERFORMANCE DISCREPANCIES

The clinical history of all the Wechsler scales is replete with various interpretations of the discrepancies between a child's Verbal and Performance IQ scores. In general, however, attempts to use the WISC-R Verbal–Performance IQ score discrepancies to distinguish between both the presence or absence of brain dysfunction and between right- and left-sided lesions have not proven to be successful (Hynd, Obrzut, and Obrzut, 1981; Sattler, 1982).

Large Verbal–Performance discrepancies have frequently been associated with possible brain damage; differences larger than 25 points are considered suggestive of neurological dysfunction (Holroyd & Wright, 1965). Black (1974) reported an index of neurologial impairment to be significantly related to the absolute magnitude of the WISC Verbal–Performance discrepancy and also discovered larger differences in children with documented brain damage than in children with suspected neurological impairment or in normal individuals. Black concluded that differences exceeding 15 points may be predictive of dysfunction. However, Bortner, Hertzig, and Birch (1972) found the Verbal–Performance discrepancies of brain-damaged children to be comparable to those differences found in normal children. Also, sizable Verbal–Performance IQ score differences can be caused by a variety of factors other than neurological dysfunction (Simenson and Sutherland, 1974). Data presented by Kaufman (1979) indicate that Verbal–Performance differences as large as 17 points cannot be considered to be outside the range of statistical normal limits.

The literature concerning Verbal–Performance differences is replete with contradictory findings concerning the relationship of Verbal–Performance differences to organic impairment. The lack of definitive studies appears to be a result of the difficulty in finding children with well-localized brain

TABLE 8-1 Verbal–Performance IQ Score Differences in Normal Children

Size of V-P difference	Percentage of children
9	48
10	43
11	39
12	34
13	31
14	28
15	24
16	22
17	18
18	16
19	14
20	12
21	10
22	8
23	7
24	6
25	5
26	4
27	3
28–30	2
31–33	1
34+	<1

Adapted from Kaufman (1979).

lesions and in obtaining refined neurological criterion information (Reed, 1976). It should be noted that much the same situation exists within the adult literature (see Matarazzo, 1972). Given the contradictory nature of the current literature, it is reasonable to state that Verbal–Performance discrepancies should not be used as a means of inferring neurological dysfunction unless there is convincing evidence available from other test data and observations.

Despite the cautions noted above, it can be said that Verbal–Performance IQ differences can be of some importance in the assessment of possible presence of brain dysfunction. The relationship between Verbal and Performance IQ score differences can still provide the clinician working with children important information about the behavioral consequences of brain damage for individuals, particularly when the WISC-R is used in conjunction with tests of sensorimotor functioning, language abilities, and visual-spatial abilities (all of these are discussed in detail in the following chapters).

In cases of documented brain damage [by computed tomography (CT) scan, medical history, etc.], the WISC-R scales can be used to assess the cognitive sequelae of the neurological impairment as well as identify adaptive deficits that may require more detailed analysis through a complete neuropsychological evaluation. If the Verbal IQ is significantly lower than the Performance IQ (by 12–15 or more points), the possibility of a language impairment should be considered (Sattler, in press). Careful analysis of the child's verbal responses to the Comprehension, Vocabulary, and Similarities subtests can help to determine possible language dysfunction. The clinician should be alert to signals of language disturbance such as difficulties in naming, word finding, comprehending instructions or specific subtest items, and so on. Responses to the Arithmetic and Digit Span subtests can offer clues as to the presence of problems in maintaining focused attention, concentration deficits, and the child's ability to deal effectively with numbers.

When Performance IQ scores exceed the Verbal IQ score by roughly the same amount, the possibility of impaired visual-perceptual functioning should be considered. Again, a careful analysis of the child's quantitative and qualitative performance can provide important information as to the presence of dysfunction. Poor performance on the Block Design, Object Assembly, and Picture Arrangement subtests may be the function of impaired visual-spatial, constructional, or perceptual organizational skills.

In summary, a large Verbal–Performance IQ score difference in isolation, regardless of direction, is not evidence of brain dysfunction. Rather, it can be used as an index through which hypotheses can be generated for further investigation through consideration of the qualitative features of a child's subtest performance, as well as behavioral observations of the child.

WECHSLER SUBTESTS AS SCREENING DEVICES

Each of the subtests of the WISC-R evaluates a number of different cognitive functions, with certain subtests being somewhat more specific than others. No single subtest has been designed to assess specifically one unique cognitive function to the exclusion of all other cognitive abilities. However, the knowledge of specifically what neuropsychological abilities each WISC-R subtest measures can be of assistance to the clinician attempting to determine if neurologically based impairment is present. The interpretive suggestions discussed in this section are not meant to be, nor are they offered as, diagnostic rules. Rather they have been listed to serve as starting points for developing and potentially testing clinical hypotheses. Any set of hypotheses generated from subtest scores needs to be integrated and confirmed or negated with hypotheses developed from qualitative features of the child's performance, and the results of other specialized assessment measures in conjunction with the child's clinical history and other pertinent information that is available.

A full description of each of the individual WISC-R subtests is beyond the scope of this book and our presumption is that the reader is familiar with the Wechsler scales. For those who are interested, detailed subtest descriptions can be found in a number of sources (e.g., Sattler, 1982, Gabel, Oster, and Butnik, 1986). What follows is a brief notation of what each of the WISC-R subtests appears to assess as well as other influences that may directly impact on a child's performance on any given subtest.

The *Information* subtest assesses the child's fund of general factual knowledge as well as verbal comprehension and long-term memory (Kaufman, 1979). This subtest is also influenced by a number of factors such as the child's interests, academic environment, cultural opportunities at home, and the richness of the child's early environment.

The *Similarities* subtest was designed to measure logical abstractive, categorical thinking. Kaufman (1979) has identified this subtest as involving verbal comprehension, and Bannatyne (1974) has noted that verbal conceptualization is an integral factor in the subtest. The Similarities subtest is also likely to be influenced by the child's outside reading.

The *Arithmetic* subtest of the WISC-R assesses computational skills as well as freedom from distractibility, verbal comprehension, sequencing, acquired knowledge, and memory (Kaufman, 1979). It can be highly influenced by the child's attention span and anxiety. In addition, Arithmetic performance can be detrimentally influenced by distractibility, the child's academic learning history, and the child's ability to work under time pressure. Since this subtest is unusually subject to outside influences, it is one of the poorest indicators of brain dysfunction.

The *Vocabulary* subtest has been designed to measure the child's word knowledge and language development. It has also been identified as tapping verbal comprehension (Kaufman, 1979), verbal conceptualization and acquired knowledge (Bannatyne, 1974), and general cognition (Guilford, 1967) as well as fund of information, learning ability, long-term memory, verbal concept formation, verbal expression, and degree of abstract thinking. A child's performance on this subtest is likely to be influenced by his cultural opportunities at home, interests, outside reading, richness of early environment, and school learning (Kaufman, 1979).

The *Comprehension* subtest is a measure of the child's ability to evaluate and use past experiences and can be viewed as a demonstration of practical information. Other abilities that influence performance on this test include verbal comprehension and conceptualization, evaluation, common sense (i.e., cause–effect relationships), social judgment, verbal expression, and verbal reasoning. Development of a "conscience" or moral sense as well as cultural opportunities at home impact on the child's performance.

The *Digit Span* subtest, the last of the verbal subtests, assesses short-term auditory memory as well as freedom from distractibility (Kaufman, 1979), sequencing skills (Bannatyne, 1974), facility with numbers, and mental alertness. As is the case with the Arithmetic subtest, performance on the Digit Span subtest can be unduly influenced by anxiety, distractibility, and attention span.

The *Picture Completion* subtest was designed to assess visual alertness as well as visual recognition and identification. As such this subtest, to some degree, measures long-term visual memory. Kaufman (1979) has noted that, via factor analysis, the subtest appears to involve primarily visual organization, and secondarily, verbal comprehension. Other areas of cognitive functioning tapped by the Picture Completion subtest include general spatial skills (Bannatyne, 1974), cognition and evaluation (Guilford, 1967). The clinician should be aware, however, that the subtest is highly subject to a number of other influences including cognitive style (i.e., field dependence versus field independence), the ability to respond when uncertain, the child's concentration, and the effects of working under time pressures.

The next subtest of the Performance subtests, *Picture Arrangement*, purports to measure temporal sequencing and time concepts in general, as well as the child's ability to anticipate consequences. In addition, the subtest is heavily dependent on perceptual organization and verbal comprehension (Kaufman, 1979), convergent production and evaluation (Guilford, 1967), integrated brain functioning, planning ability, nonverbal reasoning, social judgment, visual perception and organization of meaningful stimuli, and the ability to distinguish essential from nonessential detail (Kaufman, 1979). Other influences that can impact on the child's performance include the child's susceptibility to stress imposed by time limits, creativity, and, not surprisingly given the nature of the test, the child's exposure to comic strips.

The *Block Design* subtest assesses the child's nonverbal concept formation, spatial visualization, and the ability to analyze a whole and break it up into its components parts. Kaufman (1979) has found that this subtest loads heavily on his perceptual organization factor. Bannatyne (1974) noted that the Block Design subtest strongly involves spatial abilities whereas Guilford (1967) has found that cognition and evaluation are important for adequate performance on this test. Other skills that have been found to be involved include integrated brain functioning, visual perception, and synthesis of abstract stimuli.

The *Object Assembly* subtest of the WISC-R is a measure of the child's capacity for anticipation of relationships among parts, as well as his ability to benefit from sensory-motor feedback, and his mental flexibility. As with most of the other subtests in the Performance Scales, the Object Assembly subtest also involved perceptual organization (Kaufman, 1979), spatial skills

(Bannatyne, 1974), and cognition and evaluation (Guilford, 1967). It is subject to the influence of the child's ability to work under time constraints, experience with puzzles, and cognitive style.

Coding, both parts A and B, measures a number of skills including the ability to follow directions, clerical speed and accuracy, psychomotor speed, and short-term visual memory. Kaufman (1979) has found that a significant factor in this subtest is freedom from distractibility. Sequencing ability also was found to be important (Bannatyne, 1974), as were evaluation and convergent production (Guilford, 1967). Other abilities that are likely to be assessed, at least in part, by this subtest involve facility with numbers on part B, learning skills, paper and pencil skills, visual perception of abstract stimuli, visual-motor coordination, and the ability of the child to reproduce models. Performance on Coding is also very much subject to the child's general level of anxiety, distractibility, and his ability to work efficiently under time pressure.

The *Mazes* subtest of the Wisc-R was designed to assess the child's ability to follow a visual pattern as well as to assess the foresight of the child. It loads heavily on Kaufman's (1979) perceptual organization factor. Bannatyne (1974) reported that the test requires spatial ability, and Guilford (1967) noted that the subtest involves cognition. Other skills necesary for good performance on Mazes include planning ability, nonverbal reasoning, visual-motor coordination, paper and pencil skills, and integrated brain functions. A child's experience in solving mazes will influence performance, his ability to respond when uncertain of the correct response, and his overall responsiveness to time pressures.

EFFECTS OF BRAIN DYSFUNCTION ON WISC-R PERFORMANCE

The Information, Vocabulary, and Comprehension subtests are generally considered to be the least affected by acute brain dysfunction, except in those cases where the injury to the child has resulted in an aphasic-like disorder. For this reason, the child's scores on these subtests may provide an estimate of the child's premorbid level of functioning (Sattler, in press). In circumstances where performance on these subtests is impaired, a number of possible cognitive dysfunctions must be considered. Each of the subtests is highly dependent on intact language functioning throughout the child's development.

Deficits in verbal abstractive reasoning are likely to be seen on the Similarities subtest. In some instances, brain injury may lead to extremely concrete responses such as "an orange and a banana are not alike because one is yellow and the other is not." More often, however, the clinician is likely to receive responses that are somewhat more concrete than would be expected given the child's known (or estimated) premorbid level of functioning (e.g., an orange and a banana are alike because they taste good"). In these cases, it is extremely important that the clinician would have obtained as much premorbid information as possible from the child's parents, school, and interview.

Performance on the Digit Span subtest will sometimes reveal deficits in attention (Golden, 1981). Many clinicians attempt to use the Digit Span subtest as a measure of short-term auditory memory; however, because this subtest can be so heavily influenced by problems in attention and concentration as well as by anxiety and how the child is feeling on the day of testing, it is not advisable to do so. Large differences between the Digits Forward and Digits Backwards sections of the subtest can also be pathognomonic of brain dysfunction (Golden, 1981). Such differences may be indicative of a loss of flexibility or an inability to mentally manipulate the digits.

Sattler (1982) has noted that poor performance on the Arithmetic subtest may reveal deficient cognitive reasoning processes. When testing-of-limits procedures are employed here, the clinician can obtain useful information about sequencing, writing skills, and mastery of basic arithmetic processes. It must be remembered, however, that it is extremely important to take into consideration the child's reaction to this test (Golden, 1979). Many individuals, both adult and child, will react quite dramatically to this subtest, stating that they are unable to do arithmetic problems. Thus, an unusually low score on Arithmetic may not be very useful in identifying possible dysfunction. Low scores on this subtest that are not attributable to "math anxiety" or some other emotional response to the subtest may reflect a variety of organic problems. Generally, left hemisphere injuries will result in lower scores (Golden, 1979); however, since this subtest involves such a wide range of skills, low scores may result from almost any form of injury.

Of all the Wechsler Performance scale subtests, Picture Completion is probably the least sensitive to the effects of brain injury. Because of this, in cases where serious left hemisphere damage has occurred, performance on this subtest may represent the best single estimate of the child's premorbid functional status (Golden, 1981). Sattler (in press) notes that the subtest is occasionally sensitive to visual difficulties. If the child has a defect in his visual fields, responses such as "nothing is missing" may be given. Visual agnosia can result in the child completely misidentifying the stimulus picture. If an expressive language disturbance is present, the child may give the clinician an incorrect verbal response while simultaneously pointing to the location of the correct missing part.

Deficits in serial ordering or sequencing may result in poor performance on the Picture Arrangement subtest. Children with brain dysfunction may leave the cards in the order in which they were set out or may move them only minimally. Such behavior may reflect marked deficits in attention and concentration or generalized cognitive impairment. The clinician should be aware that Picture Arrangement generally is not very sensitive to brain dysfunction. Golden (1981) notes that performance on this subtest can be affected by damage to the right frontal areas and may be poorer than other Performance subtests in certain left hemisphere injuries that disrupt social or verbal skills.

Visual-spatial difficulties are often revealed through poor performance on the Block Design subtest. Observation of the child's performance on this subtest, perhaps more than the others on the WISC-R, is extremely important as it can reveal much information about the child's visual-spatial perceptual functioning. It is important to note whether the child has difficulty in bringing the parts together to form a whole, if there is fumbling or angulation difficulty, and the accuracy of the reproduction (Sattler, 1982). Breaks in the 2 × 2 or 3 × 3 block configuration may be indicative of visual-spatial processing problems. In addition, difficulties encountered by the child on this subtest may reflect the presence of construction dyspraxia which can be confirmed in other portions of the testing. Brain injury of many types can affect performance on the Block Design subtest, particularly injuries to the posterior portion of either hemisphere (Golden, 1981).

Performance on Object Assembly can also reveal visual-perceptual deficits. Again, it is important for the clinician to pay special attention to the types of errors the child makes. Of the subtest items failed, a distinction should be made as to whether the item(s) required appreciation of contour and edge alignment for success (e.g., the doll or horse items) or appreciation of internal detail and contour (e.g., the car or profile items). In some cases, the child will be able to identify what the item is supposed to be but will be unable to successfully complete the construction. Such information can be useful both diagnostically and prescriptively.

The Coding subtest can offer the clinician information about the child's sequencing skills, visual-motor functioning, and new learning ability. In addition, symbol perseveration or rotation as well as extreme caution or a very slow speed may signal a variety of visual processing deficits.

A poorer than expected performance on the Mazes subtest of the WISC-R can be indicative of a deficit in visual-motor coordination, flexibility, or visual-perceptual skills in general. As such, performance on this test is subject to a wide variety of brain impairment.

The clinician should bear in mind that a child's performance on intelligence tests in general, and on each of the subtests briefly discussed here, is likely to be multidetermined. For example, the written responses on the WISC-R Coding subtest are the end product of the integrations of a number of functions including visual, perceptual, oculomotor, fine manual motor, and mental abilities. Consequently, it is difficult for the generalist to determine which specific factor or combination of factors is responsible for the deficits seen during the testing. This can only be done by separately ruling out each of the suspected deficits in each of the possible functional areas related to the performance in any given subtest. Generally, this can be accomplished only through a thorough neuropsychological evaluation.

It must be emphasized that, as a test for the presense of organic dysfunction, the WISC-R is really not sensitive enough to be used in isolation. When used in combination with other tests that assess other functions, the WISC-R can be useful as a screening device; however, in a large number of instances, the WISC-R is not diagnostically accurate enough to be used in the differentiation of brain-damaged versus non–brain-damaged groups of children.

9
The Kaufman Assessment Battery for Children

The Kaufman Assessment Battery for Children (K-ABC; Kaufman and Kaufman, 1983) is a comparatively new and rather innovative measure of intelligence and achievement in children. It has been designed to test children between the ages of $2\frac{1}{2}$ and $12\frac{1}{2}$. The K-ABC is one of the few test batteries for children that was developed within the context of a strong theoretical base. It has been rigorously developed and well-standardized. The resulting test battery purports to be able to understand and measure intellectual functioning in children in a way that is different from other tests such as the WISC-R and Stanford-Binet Intelligense Test-Revised and also to measure academic achievement separately. In addition, the K-ABC also was designed to facilitate educational planning for the child. As such, the K-ABC offers some potential as a device that may be used by the generalist in such a way as to screen for the presence of cognitive dysfunction in children. Since the K-ABC is a relatively new testing device, we will devote some space to a discussion of the theories that underlie the battery as well as brief descriptions of the component parts.

THEORETICAL BASIS OF THE K-ABC

The portion of the K-ABC designed to assess intellectual functioning in children is divided into two distinct, but interrelated scales, *Sequential Processing* (i.e., manipulating material one item at a time in a determined order) and *Simultaneous Processing* (dealing with a number of pieces of information simultaneously so that the information is integrated and synthesized to form an appropriate outcome). Whereas the majority of tests of intellectual functioning, most particularly the Wechsler scales, tend to be content-oriented, this is, defined by the content of the stimuli, the K-ABC was developed so as to be process-oriented, focusing on whether the stimulus materials are dealt with one at a time or simultaneously, regardless of the item content (Kaufman and Kaufman, 1983).

Much research can be found in the literature concerning the existence of the two processing styles that underlie the K-ABC. The majority of the evidence for the K-ABC's theoretical basis comes from three primary sources: (1) research performed by cognitive and experimental psychologists in a laboratory setting; (2) factor analytical work performed by Das and his colleagues in attempting to partially validate the writings of A. R. Luria concerning functioning in the fronto-temporal versus occipital-parietal regions of the brain; and (3) research performed primarily with patients who have undergone the split-brain surgical procedure or with patients with unilateral brain damage in whom the specialized functions of the right and left hemispheres of the brain are investigated (Kaufman and Kaufman, 1983).

Each of the items that comprise the *Sequential Processing* scales presents a problem that the child must solve by arranging the stimuli in some form of serial order or sequence. In other words, each idea is related both linearly and temporally to the preceding one. While short-term memory is assessed to some degree in each task, the primary and uniting process for each item is the sequential handling of the stimuli, the method of presentation, or the response mode, regardless of the content of the item. Kaufman and Kaufman (1983) note that the ability to process material in sequential order is highly related to a number of common, school-related tasks such as memorization of lists of spelling words, number facts, and letter–sound associations. In addition, sequential processing can directly impact on the learning of grammatical relationships and rules, on comprehension of the chronology of historical events, and on application of the proper step-by-step method for numerous arithmetic operations. Difficulties in sequential processing may, therefore, have an impact on word attack skills in reading as well as on the child's ability to break a math problem into its component parts.

In contrast, the test items that compose the *Simultaneous Processing* scale are ones that are spatial and organizational in character. The stimulus material presented to the child must be integrated and synthesized simultaneously to yield the desirable solution. The mode of processing is accomplished by processing several bits of information at once rather than in a step-by-step fashion as is found in sequential problem solving. Thus, the ability to form gestalts is a necessary ability, particularly for those tasks that are primarily perceptual in nature (e.g., extracting meaning from pictures, learning the shapes of numbers and letters, etc.). Simultaneous processing also is closely related to a number of higher level cognitive processes since higher level intellectual functions require the ability to integrate information from a variety of sources, many of which may be disparate (Kaufman and Kaufman, 1983). Children with deficient simultaneous processing abilities are likely to demonstrate difficulties in comprehension of the main ideas of stories or the meaning of difficult paragraphs. Such individuals are unlikely to be able to learn efficiently more complex mathematical principles that require that the underlying meaning of numerical relationships be fully understood (Kaufman and Kaufman, 1983).

Both direct and indirect empirical evidence for the existence of a sequential-simultaneous processing dichotomy has been found within the field of cognitive psychology through the investigation of attention, basic perceptual processes, and memory (e.g., Atkinson and Shiffrin, 1968; Beller, 1970; Cohen, 1972). Simultaneous and sequential processing as defined by Luria (1966) has been investigated by Das, Kirby, and Jarman (1975, 1979). These researchers found, through a series of factor analytic studies, the consistent emergence of simultaneous and successive (sequential) factors.

THE K-ABC SUBTESTS

The K-ABC is composed of 16 subtests that assess a wide range of cognitive capabilities. It has been designed to test children ranging in age from $2\frac{1}{2}$ through $12\frac{1}{2}$ years. The average administration time ranges from about 45 minutes in preschool children to about 75 minutes for older children. The battery yields standard scores with a mean of 100 and a standard deviation of 15, much the same as the Wechsler scales. Four global measures are derived: Sequential Processing, Simultaneous Processing, a Mental Processing composite score, and an (academic) Achievement score. Of particular note is the availability of supplementary sociocultural normative data. In addition, the K-ABC has a special *Nonverbal Scale* composed of selected subtests that can be administered in pantomime, with motor responses, to permit a useful evaluation of the intellectual capabilities of hearing impaired, non–English-speaking, and speech- and language-disordered children.

Magic Window

This subtest is part of the simultaneous processing scale and has been designed to assess the ability of the child to identify and name an object whose picture is rotated behind a narrow slit so that only a portion of the picture is exposed to the child at any one time. The subtest was developed based on the experimental tasks of temporal and spatial abilities by Jarman and Nelson (1980).

In terms of cognitive functioning, the subtest assesses complex sequential integration of spatial information. Deficits in this ability are likely to lead to lowered scores. Other abilities that may impact on the child's performance include attention to essential visual detail, early language development, short-term visual memory spatial ability, and visual perception of meaningful stimuli (Kaufman and Kaufman, 1983).

Facial Recognition

This simultaneous processing scale subtest measures the child's ability to attend closely to one or two faces from a brief exposure and correctly identify the faces seen in a group photograph. Facial recognition has been found to be a highly useful tool in investigating the differential functioning of the two cerebral hemispheres (e.g., Benton, 1980). The subtest requires the capacity to maintain focused attention and is highly subject to distractibility and anxiety. It assesses visual search and scanning ability as well as facial perception and recognition.

The Facial Recognition subtest is only in the preschool portion of the K-ABC. The authors note that the underlying functions of facial recognition shift from a simultaneous processing task to one that is sequential in nature around the ages of 5–6 years. Further, Kaufman and Kaufman (1983) report that this is consistent with current theories of perceptual development (e.g., Braine, 1972) as well as with the results of studies investigating the neuropsychological aspects of face recognition (Sergent and Bindra, 1981).

Hand Movements

The Hand Movements subtest measures the ability of the child to copy the exact sequence of taps on a table with the fist, palm, or side of the hand as performed by the examiner. It is a portion of the sequential processing scale. This task is based on one developed by Luria (1966) and attempts to assess visual-motor functioning (Kaufman and Kaufman, 1983). Good concentration and attention are important to successful performance.

Although part of the sequential processing scale on the K-ABC, the Hand Movements subtest becomes a type of measure of simultaneous processing in children 5 years of age and older. This occurs because—with cognitive development—the child begins to employ a mediating strategy such as organizing the successive stimuli into a pattern to facilitate later repetition. As such, the nature of the task changes for the child into one that requires what Luria (1966) refers to as dynamic motor organization.

Gestalt Closure

This subtest is a portion of the Simultaneous Processing scale and assesses the child's ability to mentally "fill in the gaps" in a partially completed drawing and to name what is depicted. The test was developed from a series of tests of gestaltic completion by Street (1931). Closure ability requires that the child identify a complete figure based on incomplete visual information (Wasserstein, Weiss, Rosen, Gerstman, and Costa, 1980) and is a reliable measure of right hemisphere processing (Kaufman, 1979). It requires perceptual flexibility and alertness. Performance on this subtest can be impaired by a tendency toward perseveration, a field-dependent cognitive style, or the inability to respond when uncertain (Kaufman and Kaufman, 1983).

Number Recall

Number Recall measures the ability of the child to repeat in sequence a series of numbers spoken by the examiner. Obviously, this subtest is part of the sequential processing scale. It requires a good attention span on the part of the child. Performance on this subtest can easily be influenced by distractibility as well as anxiety. The task requires adequate functioning in auditory short-term memory, facility with numbers, and the ability to reproduce an auditory model (Kaufman and Kaufman, 1983).

Unlike the Digit Span subtest of the WISC-R, the Number Recall portion of the K-ABC assesses only digits forward, an ability that has consistently been shown to be a strong measure of sequential processing ability (Das, Kirby, and Jarman, 1975, 1979). Repetition of digits is a measure that has been used for several decades and was included in Binet and Simon's (1905) original intelligence test. Although most assessment devices also assess the backward digit span, research has demonstrated that it is a function of a set of cognitive abilities different from the forward digit span (Jensen and Figueroa, 1975). In addition, Costa (1975) and Weinberg, Diller, Gerstman, and Schulman (1972) have demonstrated that the different digit spans (forward vs. backward) have distinct neurological bases.

Triangles

This subtest, which is a part of the Simultaneous processing scale, assesses the child's facility at assembling numerous identical rubber triangles (blue on one side and yellow on the reverse) to match a stimulus pattern. Efficient performance on the task requires the use of a systematic strategy for mentally breaking down the model design into its component parts as well as a certain amount of cognitive flexibility in problem solving. Good visual-motor coordination, nonverbal concept formation, and spatial ability are also needed on this task.

The Triangles subtest was developed based on Kohs' Block Design Test (1927) which has been the model of all subsequently used block design tasks (e.g., Goldstein, 1948; Wechsler, 1939, 1955, 1974, 1981). This type of task has generally been considered to be a good measure of right hemisphere functioning (Lezak, 1983; Reitan, 1974).

Word Order

This sequential processing task involves the child having to point to silhouettes of common objects in the same order as they were named by the examiner, both with and without interference. It assesses a wide range of functions including attention, concentration, mental flexibility, the ability to comprehend and follow instructions, and the ability to generate a strategy for recalling the stimulus material without rehearsal. It involves both visual and verbal short-term memory as well as serial recall functions.

Word Order is an adaptation of a task developed by Luria (1966) to assess higher level cognitive functions based in the left temporal region of the brain in adults. Certain types of language disorders result in difficulty in repetition of words or series of words under interference conditions. The Word Order subtest can be sensitive to both developmental and acquired language disorders in children. The clinician must use caution in interpretation of performance on this subtest, however, because the subtest can be very much subject to distractibility, short-term memory problems (both verbal and nonverbal), anxiety, basic verbal comprehension, and deficits in visual perception.

Matrix Analogies

The Matrix Analogies subtest is part of the simultaneous processing scale and measures the child's ability to select a picture or design that best completes a 2 × 2 visual analogy. It requires cognitive flexibility, attention to essential visual detail, the ability to distinguish essential from nonessential detail, perceptual integrity, intact spatial abilities, and visual organizational ability in the absence of motor activity. The capacity to adopt a systematic strategy for inferring the nature of the analogy for each abstract item will assist the child's performance.

Matrix Analogies is similar in nature to the Raven's Progressive Matrices (Raven, 1956, 1960); however, the easy items in the Raven's Matrices do not require analogic reasoning abilities. Rather, those items depend more on pattern completion and other visual-spatial skills. Because the subtest requires that the child determine the analogy, this task can be considered to be more of a right hemisphere task (Springer and Deutsch, 1981). The K-ABC is one of the few devices for the assessment of global cognitive functioning available that assesses analogic reasoning.

Spatial Memory

This subtest, a part of the simultaneous processing scale, measures the child's ability to recall the locations of pictures randomly arranged on a page. The task requires that the child have intact visual immediate memory as well as normal spatial localization functioning. The child's performance will likely be increased if she is capable of developing a strategy for dealing with organizing the visual stimuli. In addition, cognitive flexibility becomes important when the stimulus grid changes from a 3×3 to a 3×4 grid. Kaufman and Kaufman (1983) note that performance on the subtest can be disrupted by distractibility, anxiety, and a field-dependent cognitive style. Gordon (1983) reports that localization tasks such as that used in this subtest are sensitive to right-hemisphere dysfunction. Performance on this task can be influenced by the child's general organizational capacity, her ability to reproduce a model, and a more specific visual-organizational ability.

Photo Series

In a manner similar to the WISC-R Picture Arrangement subtest, Photo Series measures the ability of the child to organize a random array of photographs illustrating an event and order them in proper sequence. It is a portion of the simultaneous processing scale despite the sequential nature of the task. To perform well, a child must have intact concentration, a nonimpulsive cognitive style, and the ability to develop a systematic strategy for evaluating and organizing the visual stimuli. An appreciation of time concepts is also important, as are the ability to anticipate consequence and a common-sense understanding of basic cause-and-effect relationships. Unlike the Picture Arrangement subtest of the WISC-R, the stimulus sets in Photo Series often do not have a social context and the subtest, in general, is not as dependent on verbal mediation as is Picture Arrangement. Other skills that can impact directly on a child's performance on this subtest include attention to essential visual detail, reasoning, visual organization without motor activity, and the ability to synthesize part-to-whole relationships.

Expressive Vocabulary

This subtest is one of the portions of the K-ABC that is a part of the Achievement Scale and assesses the ability to state correctly the name of objects in photographs. This subtest is a direct adaptation of the Picture Vocabulary subtest of the Stanford-Binet Intelligence Test, using photos instead of line drawings. The cognitive functions tapped by this subtest (i.e., verbal expression based on recognition) appear to be subserved by the left frontal regions of the brain (Hartlage and Telzrow, 1983). Performance on this subtest is a function of environmental opportunity, education, the child's interests, and alertness to the environment. Early language development, general fund of information, long-term memory, verbal concept formation, word knowledge, and visual perception of meaningful stimuli are all cognitive abilities and skills that can influence a child's score. Since performance on the Expressive Vocabulary subtest is so highly dependent on a variety of mental processes, poor performance is unlikely to be highly useful on its own in the identification of suspected brain impairment.

Faces and Places

In this achievment scale subtest, the child is required to identify and name the famous person, fictional character, or well-known place in the picture shown to the child. In essence, Faces and Places is a measure of the child's factual learning and general information acquisition from different aspects of her environment. It differs from many other achievement-oriented tests in that it assesses functions that are not highly verbal in nature (Kaufman and Kaufman, 1983). As the visual stimuli of the subtest and required verbal response from the child require integrated brain functioning, it can be viewed as somewhat of a global functioning measure. In addition, Kaufman and Kaufman (1983) note that the subtest offers the opportunity for the visual learner to demonstrate her acquired knowledge. It is unclear as to whether the functions that underlie Faces and Places represent right or left hemisphere functioning. Sergent and Bindra (1981) reported that familiar face identification requires concurrent right and left hemisphere processing whereas other investigators feel that this function is subserved primarily by the right hemisphere (Levine and Koch-Weser (1982).

The child's performance on the Faces and Places subtest is a function of the richness of her early environmente, alertness to the environment, cultural opportunities at home, interested outside reading, exposure to television, and school learning. In addition, it requires intact long-term memory, primarily simultaneous mental processing, verbal perception, and verbal expression (Kaufman and Kaufman, 1983).

Arithmetic

The Arithmetic subtest, of course, is part of the Achievement scale of the K-ABC and measures the child's ability to identify numbers, count, perform various computations, and demonstrate a general understanding of mathematical concepts. It requires integrated brain functioning. As is the case with other tests of immediate recall, performance here can be impaired by distractibility, anxiety, and a short attention span.

Riddles

Another Achievement scale subtest, Riddles assesses the ability of the child to infer the name of a concept, either concrete or abstract, when given several clues. Good performance on the subtest requires that the child have the capacity to focus on all pertinent attributes of the concept rather than attending to only a single feature. It is also necessary that the child be able to integrate sequentially presented auditory-verbal stimuli, infer concepts, and classify material logically. Distractibility, a tendency toward perseveration, and an impulsive response style may all act to lower the child's performance.

Reading/Decoding

The Reading/Coding subtest of the K-ABC assesses the ability to identify letters as well as to read and pronounce words. It is similar in many ways to the Reading subtest of the Wide Range Achievement Test (Jastak and Wilkinson, 1984). The subtest measures the skills of decoding, letter naming, word attack skills, word recognition, and pronunciation. Other important functions involved in the child's performance on this subtest include basic achievement, early language development, long-term memory, both sequential and simultaneous processing, visual perception, and verbal expression.

Reading/Understanding

The last of the Achievement scale subtests, this one measures the child's ability to demonstrate reading comprehension by acting out commands that are presented to the child in sentences. In other words, the child is required to perform gestures or movements to show the meaning of what he has just read, thereby avoiding confounding by impaired short-term memory or impaired visual perception of nonverbal stimuli. The use of a nonverbal response mode requires integrated brain functioning, since reading is considered to be primarily a left hemisphere task and gestural communication is thought to be a right hemisphere function (Springer and Deutsch, 1981). Adequate performance on the Reading/Understanding subtest is highly dependent on richness of early environment, alertness to the environment, cultural opportunities at home, outside reading, and school learning. Verbal concept formation, basic reading skills, and both simultaneous and sequential mental processing are also important factors that contribute to the child's performance.

THE K-ABC AS A SCREENING INSTRUMENT FOR BRAIN DYSFUNCTION

The authors of the K-ABC stress the utility of the battery with virtually all special (exceptional) populations of children. This is meant to include children who are learning-disabled, behaviorally disordered, mentally retarded, hearing impaired, physically handicapped, and gifted. Since the K-ABC is a new assessment device, there have been few, if any, research investigations that have addressed the validity of the above claims or the utility of the battery as a screening device. Nonetheless, some general comments concerning its use are appropriate.

The K-ABC was developed through the use of strong empirical research and has a sound theoretical basis. All of the processing subtests in the battery have been derived from existing tests which have demonstrated empirical validity and reliability. The majority of the subtests of the K-ABC also were derived from measures that have been shown to be effective in identifying cognitive dysfunctions in adults, if not in children.

Intuitively, then, there is a very high likelihood that the presence of cognitive dysfunction in a child will be identified by poor performance on some portions of the battery. Since there is no direct empirical support linking poor performance on a given K-ABC subtest with either localized or diffuse brain injury, the qualitive aspects of the child's performance on any given task become increasingly important and must be noted.

Cognitive functioning is differentially affected by different types and locations of brain damage (Golden, 1979). Recognition of this fact, in conjunction with the knowledge that each of the K-ABC's subtests are subject to influence by a wide range of cognitive functions not directly assessed by a specific subtest, leads to the conclusion that the K-ABC is best used as a screening device for making general statements concerning the presence or absence of brain dysfunction in a child.

Part III
ASSESSMENT INSTRUMENTS AND THEIR USES

10
Screening Tests of Perceptual, Cognitive, and Motor Functioning

A variety of instruments exist to test children and can be used as a part of a comparatively brief yet comprehensive screening of higher cognitive functions. Many of the tests that will be discussed in this chapter have been designed to assess somewhat more generalized cognitive functioning as opposed to those devices that tap fairly specific functional capabilities. Unlike the WISC-R and K-ABC, which are multiple subtest batteries, these instruments are generally single tests, some of which have several conditions.

As is the case in adults, dysfunction of higher cognitive functions in chidren is not necessarily associated with damage to a specific cortical region. Rather, higher level cognitive abilities generally are sensitive to the effects of brain damage regardless of the site of the damage. It must be remembered that higher level functions always involve an intact system for organizing perceptual information, an extensive and easily available database of learned information, integrity of cortical and subcortical interconnections, integrity of patterns that are commonly referred to as "thinking," and the capacity to process multiple mental events simultaneously.

The clinician working with children must constantly keep in mind that cognitive functioning in children in general differs significantly from that which occurs in adults. Brain damage in childhood does not produce the same pattern of deficits seen in late childhood or adult brain damage. The effects of early brain damage will be seen differentially depending on the task or test chosen and on the normal developmental pattern of performance for that task. It is likely that at different developmental levels, the same task is completed in different ways (Wilkening and Golden, 1982). Although the final behavior may be the same, the psychological processes utilized for that behavior may be entirely different. This points to the necessity that any test used be interpreted in the face of developmental information and theory.

Teuber and Rudel (1962) conducted research that emphasized that there are some tasks in which the effects of brain damage on children's behavior are not immediately apparent, although performance on the same task at a later age will give evidence of impairment. If a skill is acquired later in life, it makes little sense to assume that a task employing this skill will differentiate normal from brain-injured children prior to the normal developmental emergence of this skill. This research also supports the notion that there are behavioral similarities between brain-damaged children and adults that can be observed when appropriate test materials are used.

At the present time, there is comparatively little research indicating at what ages specific cognitive abilities emerge; however, some *rough* guidelines do exist based on the theories of Luria (1966). The approach used by Luria concerning neuropsychological development can be useful in understanding the cognitive functioning and behavior of children as he also developed a scheme for describing neurological development that was based on physiological as well as functional data. In a neuropsychological sense neurological development results from myelinizationm, dendritic and neurological growth, and the establishment of pathways among cells as well as what are likely to be unrecognized physical and biochemical events (Golden, 1981). The relationship between physical development of the cortex and psychological maturation is not, as yet, adequately understood. To identify more accurately deviant or unusual patterns of maturation, further research will be necessary.

Based on Luria's (1966) theory, there are five stages in neuropsychological development. These stages generally correspond to the emergence of functions of various cortical areas (Wilkening and Golden, 1982). The first stage involves maturation and operation of the reticular system and those structures necessary for maintaining optimum levels of arousal and attention. Generally, this system becomes mature and operational early in the first year of life, although development of this system is more closely related to the time since conception than time since birth. It is most vulnerable to damage while it is forming during the perinatal period.

Stage two occurs concurrently with the development of stage one (Wilkening and Golden, 1982). It is during this stage that the three primary sensory areas (visual, tactile, auditory) and the motor area develop. During stage three, which occurs concomitantly with the first two stages but continues through the preschool period, the unimodal association areas and the secondary areas of the cortex become functional. Skills such as coordinated movement, auditory and visual recognition and discrimination, and the association of words and objects develop. Although cross modality learning occurs here as a function of rote memory, integrative problem-solving generally does not occur.

The area of the brain responsible for integration of multimodal sensory integration (tertiary parietal cortex) is involved in stage four of development. Golden (1981) notes that this region is not thought to be active until the ages of about 5 to 8 years. This region of the brain is believed to be intimately involved in the acquisition and use of most academic skills such as reading, analogic reasoning, categorization, and so on. Most standard measures of intellectual functioning such as the Wechsler scales assess these skills.

The fifth and final stage of neuropsychological development involves the prefrontal cortex and is not thought to occur until adolescence (Wilkening and Golden, 1982). This brain region is believed to be responsible for maintaining intention and planning, the evaluation of behavior, impulse control, and cognitive flexibility.

The general clinician who is asked to evaluate the cognitive integrity of a child will typically be evaluating stage four functions. Therefore, the assessment devices discussed in this chapter, as well as the majority of those discussed throughout this book, will be evaluating the cognitive capabilities that become available to the child during stage four of neuropsychological development.

VISUAL FUNCTIONS

A variety of aspects of visual functioning can be impaired by brain injury in children. As a general rule, brain damage in a child that results in disruption of one visual function will affect a cluster of related visual functions as well. A major division in visual functions occurs between those involving verbal-symbolic material and those dealing with nonsymbolic stimuli. Other stimulus dimensions that may highlight different aspects of visual perception are the degree to which the stimulus is structured, the amount of remote and new memory involved in the task, spatial relationships, and the presence of interfering information. We will begin with tests for more basic functions such as simple perception and recognition, and proceed to higher order tasks such as visual-spatial relationships and visual-motor coordination.

Color Perception

A screening test of color perception can serve a threefold purpose in assessing children in whom cognitive dysfunction is suspected. It can identify children with congenitally defective color vision (color blindness) whose performance on tasks requiring accurate color recognition might otherwise be misinterpreted. Such knowledge will have a major impact on the clinician's overall interpretation of the child's responses to such colored material as that in the Color Sorting Test. Tests of color perception can also be used to determine the potential presence of color agnosia. Finally, a color perception screening can serve as an "ice breaker" of sorts since the task is relatively easy for most children and helps to establish rapport with the child.

Two of the most widely used tests of color perception in a standard neuropsychological assessment are the Ishihara (1964) and the Dvorine (1953) Screening Tests. Each test requires that the child view a card printed with different colored dots that form recognizable figures against a background of contrasting colored dots. All of the dots are matched for color saturation so that the child will not be influenced by the "brightness" of a particular color. Those children who truly have defective color perception, and not a problem with color agnosia (the inability to identify colors despite intact color discrimination vision), will be unable to see the stimulus figure against the background. In contrast, the child with intact color vision and a color agnosia will be able to make the necessary discriminations but may not be able to differentiate between a red ball and a blue ball.

Motor-Free Visual Perception Test

The Motor-Free Visual Perception Test (MVPT; Colarusso & Hammill, 1972) was originally designed to allow the clinician to obtain an accurate and reliable assessment of a child's basic visual-perceptual capabilities without employing a motor component as is quite common in many other measures of various aspects of visual perception. The 36 items that make up the test can be administered in about 10 minutes and require little training on the part of the examiner. The child is shown two pages of a booklet. On the top page, a single geometric shape is presented while on the bottom page a number of similar and dissimilar geometric shapes are presented with only one being exactly the same as the target shape. The child must indicate which of the alternatives is the same as the target stimulus. Scoring is objective and the resulting raw score is compared with normative data that accompanies the test. The MVPT provides two types of normative data: perceptual ages and perceptual quotients for children ranging in age from 4 to 8 years.

VISUAL RECOGNITION

Interest in visual recognition in children has grown with the rapid expansion of the knowledge of the different roles played by the hemispheres and with more precise understanding of the different functional systems within the brain. When brain damage is present or suspected, examining different aspects of visual recognition on a gross level can lead to a clearer idea of the child's status and can offer valuable information for educational planning.

Picture Recognition

Meaningful Pictures (Battersby et al., 1956) was designed to highlight asymmetrical perceptual defects. The test requires a number of colored magazine illustrations or photographs that are essentially symmetrical on either side of the median plane. Each picture is presented first as a verbal recall task in which, after a 10-second exposure, the child is asked to name and indicate the relative position of the details of the picture seen. When the recall section of the test is completed, the child is again shown the illustration and asked to describe all its details while viewing it. Card sides can then be compared for the number of responses elicited from the child. A preponderance of responses that describe one side of the picture or the other suggests the presence of lateralized visual inattention (or a lesion in the brain) on the opposite side.

Another commonly used test that can be used to assess visual recognition is the revised version of the Peabody Picture Vocabulary Test (PPVT) (Dunn & Dunn, 1981). The PPVT-R was designed primarily to assess an individual's receptive vocabulary (the PPVT-R is described in greater detail elsewhere in the book). As such it an be an effective tool for assessing both language disorders and perceptual functioning. Using a nonstandard procedure, the clinician can have the child name a number of pictures on various pages of the test booklet. Although no normative data exist for this procedure, the child's performance can give the clinician a fairly good idea as to whether a picture recognition deficit exists from which the presence of possible brain dysfunction can be inferred.

Face Recognition

Warrington and James (1967) demonstrated that there is no regular relationship between the inability to recognize familiar faces (prosopagnosia) and impaired recognition of unfamiliar faces. This has led to a separation of facial recognition tests into those that involve a memory component and those that do not. Tests of familiar facial recognition require a memory component and generally use the faces of popular figures and well-known historical figures; the memory element is one of the difficulties with this form of test. If a child performs poorly on such a test, it is difficult to determine if the primary problem involves perceptual recognition or visual memory.

To avoid this difficulty and examine the ability to recognize faces without involving memory, Benton and Van Allen (1968) developed the Test of Facial Recognition in which the individual is asked to match identical front-view photographs of an unknown person, front with side views, and front views taken under different lighting conditions. Although originally designed for use with adults, the test can readily be used with children from age five and up. For children under age 5, an alternative to the Test of Facial Recognition is the Facial Recognition subtest of the K-ABC (Kaufman and Kaufman, 1983).

An individual with problems in facial recognition usually will have right hemisphere dysfunction. The presence of a language disorder or visual field defects should not interfere significantly with visual recognition tasks (Lezak, 1983); however, facial recognition deficits do tend to occur with spatial agnosia and dyslexia, as well as with dysgraphias (problems with writing) that involve spatial disturbance (Tzavaras, Hecaen, & LeBras, 1970).

COMPLEX VISUAL FUNCTIONS

Tests of Spatial and Visuomotor Abilities

There are a large number of tests of complex visual abilities as they have long been popular as single tests of brain injury. Golden (1981) noted that this may be based on the known representation of complex spatial functions in both cerebral hemispheres. It may also be a function of the fact that it is sometimes easier to encourage the cooperation of a child on those tasks that require minimal verbal responding.

The Trail Making Test for Children

The Trail Making Test (Army Individual Test, 1944) has been used for several years as an easily administered test of visual-conceptual and visuomotor tracking for adults. As is the case for most other tests that have a large attentional component, it is extremely sensitive to the effects of brain injury (Reitan, 1958).

The children's version of the Trail Making Test was developed as part of an overall downward extension of the Halstead–Reitan Neuropsychological Battery for Adults which was started by Reitan and his colleagues at the Indiana University Medical Center in 1951. It is given in two parts, A and B (Figure 10-1). The children's version of this test is appropriate for children ages six through 14 years.

The child is asked to draw lines connecting 15 consecutively numbered circles on Part A of the test, and then is asked to connect the same number of consecutively numbered (1 through 8) and lettered ("A" through "G")

Screening Tests of Perceptual, Cognitive, and Motor Functioning

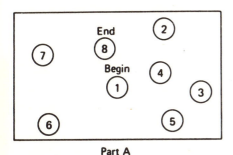 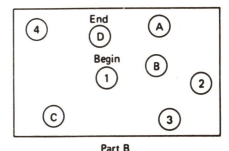

Part A   Part B

FIGURE 10-1. Practice samples of the Trail-Making Test.

circles on a second sheet by alternating between numbers and letters (Part B). The time required to complete each form of the test is recorded by the clinician as are the number of errors. Errors are pointed out to the child so that they can be corrected. The effects of error correction are reflected in the total time required to complete each section. In addition, total time to complete both parts of the test and the total number of errors can be calculated for comparison to the limited normative data that are currently available (Table 10-1).

The Trail Making Test requires immediate recognition of the symbolic significance of both letters and numbers as well as the ability to scan the page continuously to identify the next letter or number in the sequence. Flexibility in integrating the numerical and alphabetical series and completion of these requirements under the pressure of time are also an integral part of the test. Reitan and Wolfson (1985) note that it seems likely that the ability to deal with the numerical and language symbols is subserved by the functioning of the left cerebral hemisphere, that the visual scanning portion of the task necessary to perceive the spatial distribution of the stimulus material is represented by the right side of the brain, and that the speed and efficiency of performance required by the test may be generally characteristic of adequate brain functioning. Therefore, it is not surprising that the test can be a good general measure of cognitive functioning. This is particularly true for part B of the test (Teeter, 1986).

Bender Visual-Motor Gestalt Test

The Bender Visual-Motor Gestalt Test is arguably one of the oldest and most widely used tests of complex visual processing. The Bender has been used extensively throughout the world as a screening device as well as a portion of a more complete psychological test battery to assess developmental, cognitive-perceptual, and emotional problems in both children and adults.

TABLE 10-1 Trail Making Test Scores for Normal Control Subjects

		Age					
		9	10	11	12	13	14
Trails A—time	M	25.1	22.5	20.9	19.7	16.8	14.9
	SD	10.5	6.6	6.3	7.1	5.4	3.3
Trails B—time	M	54.9	52.8	40.5	38.5	30.9	31.6
	SD	22.0	26.3	15.0	16.1	7.3	10.7
Total time	M	80.0	75.3	61.4	58.2	47.7	46.1
	SD	28.1	30.4	20.3	22.7	10.3	13.0

Times are in seconds

Adapted from Klonoff, H. & Low, M. (1976). Disordered brain function in young children and early adolescents: Neuropsychological and electroencephalographic correlates. In R. M. Reitan & L. A. Davison (Eds.), *Clinical neuropsychology: Current status and applications* (pp. 121–178), Washington, D.C.; V. H. Winston & Sons. Adapted with permission.

As has been noted elsewhere, *it is also one of the most widely misused tests for determining the presence or absence of brain damage* (Berg, Franzen, and Wedding, 1987). A review of the relevant literature demonstrates that the Bender appears to have been considered as a virtual panacea among psychological tests. For instance, Hutt (1963) has noted that the test has been reported as being useful in establishing rapport with the individual being tested, assessing uneducated or culturally deprived individuals, detailing emotional conflict, predicting various aspects of academic achievement, studying intercultural differences, investigating the link between perceptual-motor behavior and a variety of personality traits, estimating intelligence, identifying juvenile delinquents, and determining whether a child has learning deficits.

Originally, the Bender was constructed as a visual-motor performance task with adult patients and as a developmental screening examination for children (Bender, 1938). The nine geometric designs (presented in Figure 10-2) used in the test were based on the work of Max Wertheimer, one of the early Gestalt psychologists. The designs consist of dots, lines, angles, and curves that form a variety of relationships. Each design is on a card that approximates the size of an enlarged index card.

The underlying principle of the Bender was that the organized whole is the primary form of perception in humans. Any loss or disruption of this integrative perception might, therefore, be indicative of some form of pathology (Gabel, Oster, & Butnik, 1986). It was originally thought that neurological injury, emotional dysfunction, or changes in intellectual functioning could significantly impact on the process of perception and reproduction of the test figures. These initial hypotheses were investigated with a variety of clinical patients who suffered from aphasia, generalized

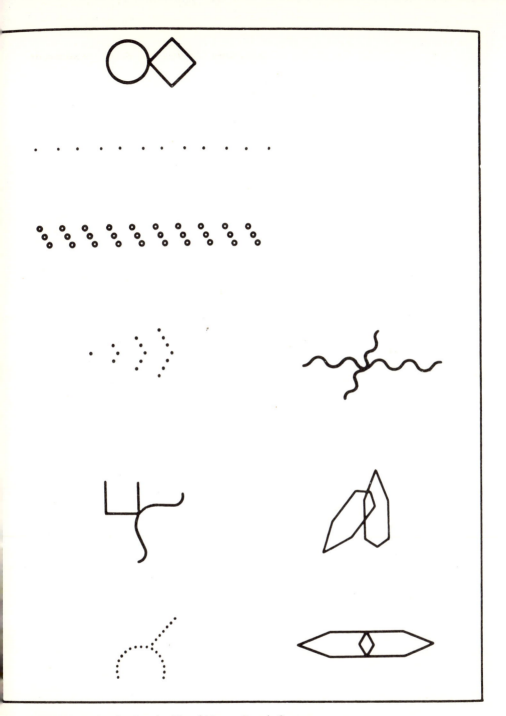

FIGURE 10-2. The Bender Visual-Motor Gestalt figures.

From Bender, L. (1938). *A visual motor gestalt test and its clinical use* (American Orthopsychiatric Association Research Monographs No. 3). Reproduced by permission.

organic brain syndrome, mental retardation, schizophrenia, manic-depressive illness, and anxiety disorders as well as in normal children (Bender, 1938).

With respect to the utility of the Bender as a measure of cortical integrity, a number of clinicians have a tendency to use the Bender, and only the Bender, to identify cortical dysfunction. This approach should be avoided since the test has *not* been shown effectively to perform this exclusive function. The danger of this use lies in the Bender's high rate of false-negative findings in uncovering general cortical dysfunction.

In using the Bender, the clinician usually provides the child with several of sheets blank paper nearby on an examining table with pencils and erasers. Typically one sheet of paper is placed before the child. She is then asked to copy each of the nine geometric figures and patterns on the paper, one at a time. After the first card (Design A) is presented to the child, she may ask as to where to draw this (and subsequent) figure(s). The clinician must allow the child to solve this problem herself, offering only minimal guidance (e.g., "Anywhere you would like," "Anywhere you think is right," "Do as well as you can," etc.) since observation of the child's planning abilities offers valuable qualitative information. Additional sheets of paper can be used by the child as needed. These either can be provided by the clinician or taken by the child if she feels they are necessary.

The drawings are than evaluated using one of several scoring systems that have been developed over the years. Each of these scoring systems has attempted to identify qualitative signs indicating brain damage. In some cases, variations of these approaches also attempt to identify emotional disorders. Some of the most popular of these scoring systems include those presented by Bender (1938), Hain (1964), Hutt (1969), Pascal and Suttell (1951).

Another highly popular system for use with children is one developed by Koppitz (1963, 1975) which provides a scoring method based on normative data collected from children ages 5 to 10. The research by Koppitz included comparisons of scores obtained from the Bender with measures of intellectual functioning and academic achievement. In one study, Koppitz (1975) found that seven errors in copying figures discriminated between good and poor students of early elementary school age. These errors included distortion of shape, rotations, substitutions of circles or dashes for dots, perseveration, part of figures not joined, three or more angles in a curve, and missing or extra angles. In addition, Koppitz established a list of 29 indicators of brain damage for the Bender (see Table 10-2) based on the type of errors made and on which specific designs the errors were made. However, there are also strong cautions that several of these signs must be present before the issue of the possible presence of brain damage can be raised.

TABLE 10-2 Koppitz' Bender Visual-Motor Gestalt Indicators of Brain Dysfunction for Children Age 5 to 10

Error type[a]	Figure	Age 5	6	7	8	9	10
1	A	x	x	x	x	x	x
	7	x	x	x	x	x	x
	8			x	x	x	x
2	6	x	x	x	x	x	x
3	6	x	x	x	x	x	x
4	A			x	x	x	x
	7				x	x	x
5	1	x	x	x	x	x	x
	3			x	x	x	x
	5					x	x
6	A	x	x	x	x	x	x
	1	x	x	x	x	x	x
	2					x	x
	3				x	x	x
	4	x	x	x	x	x	x
	5	x	x	x	x	x	x
	7			x	x	x	x
	8	x	x	x	x	x	x
7	A	x	x	x	x	x	x
	4	x	x	x	x	x	x
	6	x	x	x	x	x	x
	7			x	x	x	x
8	2			x	x	x	x
9	3		x	x	x	x	x
10	3	x	x	x	x	x	x
	5	x	x	x	x	x	x
11	1				x	x	x
	2				x	x	x
	6				x	x	x

x, Significant indicator of brain dysfunction at this age level for this figure

[a] Error types: 1, extra or missing angles; 2, angles for curves; 3, straight line for curves; 4, disproportion of parts; 5, substitution of five circles for dots; 6, rotation of design by 45 (or more) degrees; 7, failure to integrate parts; 8, omission or addition of rows of circles; 9, shape of design lost; 10, line for series of dots; 11, perseveration.

Adapted from Koppitz, E. M. (1963). *The Bender Gestalt Test for young Children.* New York: Grune & Stratton. Adapted with permission.

In its current usage, the Koppitz developmental Bender scoring system is divided into two sections—developmental age scoring and emotional indicators. As a system in evaluating cognitive maturation, the developmental scores are used to assess visual-motor functioning. Scorable errors have been divided into four general categories: shape distortion, rotation, integration difficulties, and perseveration. The total number of errors made by the child is compared to normative values that were developed by Koppitz (1963) are presented in Table 10-3.

Successful performance on the Bender requires both perceptual-motor focus and discrimination (Palmer, 1970). At the simplest level, the child must have the ability to concentrate and attend to the figure. At a more complex level, she must be able to separate the component parts of the figure and then integrate it into a unified whole, or Gestalt. A child may be able to determine that a design consists of two basic parts but may not be able to reproduce both parts (e.g., drawing two squares, instead of the circle

TABLE 10-3 Normative Data for the Koppitz Developmental Bender Scoring System

Age group (years and months)	Mean errors	Standard deviation
5–0 to 5–5	13.6	3.61
5–6 to 5–11	9.7	3.72
6–0 to 6–5	8.4	4.12
6–6 to 6–11	6.4	3.76
7–0 to 7–5	4.8	3.61
7–6 to 7–11	4.7	3.34
8–0 to 8–5	3.7	3.60
8–6 to 8–11	2.5	3.03
9–0 to 9–5	1.7	1.76
9–6 to 9–11	1.6	1.69
10–0 to 10–5	1.6	1.67
10–6 to 10–11	1.5	2.10

Distribution of Bender Scores by Grade Placement

Grade placement at beginning of year	Mean age	Mean score	Standard deviation
Kindergarten	5–4	13.5	3.61
Grade 1	6–5	8.1	4.41
Grade 2	7–5	4.7	3.18
Grade 3	8–7	2.2	2.03
Grade 4	9–8	1.5	1.88

Adapted from Koppitz, E. M. (1963). *The Bender Gestalt Test for young children.* New York: Grune & Stratton. Adapted with permission.

and square when attempting to copy Design A). Motor functioning is also incorporated in these abilities.

The child must have developed the ability to focus on a single, distinct motor movement and to be able to discriminate between movements when performing the Bender. To complete the test, the child must have reached a developmental level that allows her to hold a drawing implement, usually a pencil, without opposing movements that would impede performance. It is also important for the child to be able to choose appropriate movements that allow her to accurately reproduce the figures. Thus, age becomes an important factor in use of the Bender. Generally, although currently available scoring systems often begin at age 5, children younger than age 6 are likely to do so poorly that it becomes impossible to obtain useful clinical information from the test.

Investigators who have used the various scoring systems developed for the Bender have reported up to 70% accuracy in identifying brain-injured individuals and a hit rate of 90% in identifying normal subjects (e.g., Brilliant and Gynther, 1963; Levine & Feirstein, 1972). However, *there have been as many or more other studies using the Bender that have reported essentially negative results*. Several major review articles have leveled criticism at the Bender for its unreliability and inability to discriminate brain-injured from non–brain-injured populations (e.g., Billingslea, 1963; Canter, 1976; Tolor & Schulberg, 1963).

In general, the results of many years of research indicate that using the Bender as the sole instrument to identify brain damage allows far too wide a margin of error in clinical work. A poor score on the Bender Visual-Motor Gestalt Test may in fact indicate problems for a child; however, it does not necessarily indicate the nature of the deficit. Similarly, and perhaps more importantly, good performance on the test does not conclusively rule out the possible presence of cognitive dysfunction. For this reason, the Bender should never be used in isolation.

Raven's Coloured Progressive Matrices

Raven's Progressive Matrices were originally designed as a culture-free measure of intelligence (Raven, 1960). Although subsequent investigation has shown that the test did not meet this goal, it does appear to offer a measure of visual reasoning. The test is easy to administer and can be given with little formal training. The test is untimed and, on average, takes 15–30 minutes. It consists of 36 items, grouped into three series, plus sample items. The Coloured Progressive Matrices were designed for children ages 5 through 11 years. Each item contains a pattern with one part missing and from four to six picture inserts, one of which contains the correct pattern (see Figure 10-3). The child is instructed to point to the pattern piece she feels will complete the larger pattern. Alternatively, the child can record her response on an answer sheet.

There are two other versions of the test, the Standard Progressive Matrices and the Advanced Progressive Matrices, both of which have norms available for ages 8–65, although the advanced test should not be used with children under 11½ years. In all forms of the test, raw scores are converted to percentiles. Generally, the poorer the performance of the child, the more likely the presence of dysfunction.

Block Design Tests

Block design tests require the child to reproduce a pattern, usually using multicolored blocks. The most frequently used block tests are those that are part of the Wechsler Intelligence Scales, the Block Design subtests in the WISC-R (ages 6–16) (Wechsler, 1974), and WPPSI (ages 4–6) (Wechsler, 1967). In this task, the child is presented with a picture of a red and white design that must be constructed using from two to nine blocks, depending on which Wechsler scale is being used. The WISC-R blocks have been designed such that each block has two sides that are completely red; two sides that are completely white; and two sides that are half red and half white split along the diagonal. The WPPSI blocks are flat and have a completely red side and one that is red and white split along the diagonal. Research has shown that performance on this

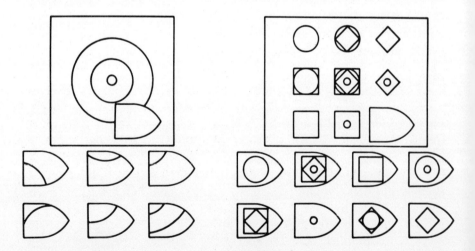

FIGURE 10-3. Examples of the Raven's Progressive Matrices Test.

task is sensitive to right hemisphere lesions (McFie, 1975); however, in children, performance on this task can be affected by dysfunction anywhere in the brain.

Judgment of Line Orientation

This test developed by Benton and his colleagues (1975) examines the ability of the child to estimate angular relationships between line segments by visually matching angled line pairs to 11 numbered radii that form a semicircle. The test includes 30 items, each of which shows a different pair of angled lines to be matched to the display cards. The test has two forms, H and V, which present the same items but in a different order. The actual test is preceded by five practice items to familiarize the child with the task. The test manual provides normative data for both adults and children. In general, individuals with left hemisphere damage tend to perform normally on the test while the presence of right hemisphere damage generally leads to poor performance, particularly if the damage is located in the posterior regions.

Puzzle Solving

The Puzzle Solving subtest of the McCarthy Scales of Children's Abilities (McCarthy, 1972) requires that the child assemble six cut-up picture puzzles that depict either a common animal or object. Each of the first two puzzles is comprised of only two pieces whereas the last puzzles are fairly complex. All items are timed with 30–120 seconds allotted depending on the complexity of the puzzle. Bonus points for rapid performance can be earned on the last three puzzles. The test was designed to be administered to children ranging in age from $2\frac{1}{2}$ to $8\frac{1}{2}$ years (as is the case with the rest of the battery). A child's ability to solve the puzzles involves basic visual perception as well as nonverbal reasoning, visual-motor coordination, and spatial relations. A child's performance that is poor when compared to the normative data supplied with the McCarthy scales can be viewed as indicative of a cognitive dysfunction; however, the specific nature and extent of the dysfunction cannot be determined from this test alone.

Pictorial Test of Intelligence—Similarities

The Similarities subtest of the Pictorial Test of Intelligence (French, 1964) is an easily administered device that is designed to tap a child's complex cognitive reasoning abilities based on visual input. A four-item visual display is presented to the child and she is asked to identify the picture that is different from the other three. For some of the items in the subtest, the discriminations are based on differences in detail such as a different number of apples on a tree. With other items, the difference is at the conceptual level (e.g., which of four food items is not a dessert food). Thus, different cognitive skills are involved for each of the types of tasks presented in the test. The examiner scores the test results and raw scores are converted to standard scores based on the available normative data which is presented in the test manual. Although the resulting standard score can be useful, a better and more clinically useful approach is for the clinician to perform an error analysis to determine the cognitive domain in which the deficit lies. Total administration time is roughly 5 minutes and the test is for children ages 2 years, 10 months to 8 years.

ITPA Visual Association Test

The Visual Association subtest of the Illinois Test of Psycholinguistic Abilities (ITPA; Kirk, McCarthy, & Kirk, 1968) is composed of two conceptually distinct sets of task demands. In the first part of the subtest, the child is presented with a visual display composed of a stimulus picture and four possible response items. The child is asked to indicate the item most closely associated with the target picture. For the second part of the subtest, the child is required to complete visual analogies. The exemplar item consists of two pictures that present an analogic relationship. On the same page, the child is presented with a target stimulus and asked to find the item among an array of four that is related to the target picture in the same way as the exemplar items are related. Administration time is typically less than 5 minutes and the test is appropriate for children from 2 years, 4 months to 10 years, 3 months of age.

Both parts of the test involve conceptual-linguistic skills; however, each part of the test requires a different level of processing. The first part of the test is easy relative to the more complex second part. The child's scoring does not reflect this comparative ease and the clinician should carefully analyze the child's performance to determine which section of the test was more difficult for the child.

AUDITORY FUNCTIONS

The verbal and nonverbal components of auditory perception appear to be functionally distinct (Milner, 1962). A number of techniques for assessing auditory functioning in children are available, a representative sample of which will be briefly discussed here. To date, neuropsychology has paid comparatively little attention to nonverbal auditory functioning. Thus, although numerous verbal tests involving audition exist, the psychological examination of the nonverbal aspects of auditory perception is limited to a few techniques.

Every evaluation provides some opportunity to evaluate the auditory perception of verbal material. When the clinician orally presents problems of judgment and reasoning, learning and memory, the opportunity also arises to informally assess the child's auditory acuity and comprehension as well as processing capacity. Significant deficits in the perception and comprehension of speech can become readily apparent quite rapidly during the course of administering most psychological tests.

If a few tasks with simple instructions requiring only motor responses or one- or two-word answers are given, subtle problems with auditory processing can easily be missed. These include difficulty in processing or retaining lengthy messages, although responses to single words or phrases may be accurate; inability to handle spoken numbers without a concomitant impairment in processing other forms of speech; an inability to process information at high levels in the auditory system when the ability to repeat them accurately remains intact; or the inability to focus and maintain attention in the presence of competing auditory information. In the absence of a primary hearing disorder, any impairment in the individual's capacity to recognize or effectively process speech may indicate a lesion in the dominant cerebral hemisphere.

When impaired auditory processing is suspected in a child, the clinician can couple an auditorily presented task with a similar test presented visually. This kind of paired testing enables the clinician to compare the functioning of both perceptual systems under similar conditions. If the child demonstrates a consistent tendency to perform better under one of the two conditions, the possibility of neurological impairment of the less efficient perceptual system exists.

Nonverbal Auditory Perception

As the majority of human behavior is organized around verbal signals, there is a potential for overlooking nonverbal auditory functions. The recognition, discrimination, and comprehension of nonsymbolic sound patterns such as music, tapping patterns, rhythms, and meaningful noises (thunder, automobile horns, sirens, etc.), are subject to impairment as much as is the perception of language sounds. Dysfunction in nonverbal auditory perception tends to be associated with brain damage in the right temporal region of the brain (Milner, 1962).

Seashore Rhythm Test

Most assessment devices for nonverbal auditory functioning use sound recordings. The Seashore Rhythm Test (Seashore, Lewis, & Saetveit, 1960) is probably the most widely used test since it was incorporated into the test battery developed by Halstead (1947). This test can be used with children age 9 years and older. The test requires that the child listen to pairs of tone groups and determine whether the tone groups in the pair are the same or different from one another. The test is scored in terms of the number of errors, a greater number of errors suggesting dysfunction. Since a component of the test assesses ability to attend and make rapid decisions, the tape should not be stopped once it is started and the child should be encouraged to keep up with the tape.

The clinician can also improvise tests for nonverbal auditory perception. The original Halstead and Wepman Aphasia Screening Test requires the patient to identify a tune ("America"). Alternatively, the child can be asked to identify any popular melody, such as "Happy Birthday." A child raised in the United States who is unable to recognize a very common and popular tune may be demonstrating an amusia suggesting possible right temporal lobe damage. The clinician also can assess which of two sounds is higher. (These sounds can be hummed or whistled.) Recognition of rhythmic patterns can be evaluated by requiring the child either to discriminate similar and different sets of rhythmic taps or to mimic patterns tapped out by the examiner.

Luria-Nebraska Neuropsychological Battery Rhythm Scale

An alternative testing procedure that can be used with children from age 8 to 12 is the Rhythm Scale of the Luria–Nebraska Battery-Children's Revision (Golden, 1987). The scale has many components of the Seashore Rhythm Test as well as other of the features noted previously. Many of the stimuli are on tape so that each child will receive essentially the same stimuli in the same manner. One added feature of this scale is that normative data are available for comparison. The scale can be administered by an experienced examiner quite easily in about 10–15 minutes. Little formal training is required to administer this scale. (This is not the case for the complete test battery.) One potential drawback in using the Rhythm scale is that the complete battery must be purchased which, although not as costly as other comprehensive neuropsychological assessment batteries, requires a substantial investment. For children older than 12 years, the adult version of the LNNB Rhythm Scale can be used.

Goldman–Fristoe–Woodcock Auditory Diagnostic Battery

The Goldman–Fristoe–Woodcock (GFW) Auditory Diagnostic Battery (Goldman, Fristoe, & Woodcock, 1974–1976) evaluates auditory discrimination skills in children. The battery is divided into three sections, each of which requires the child to point to one of two pictures that represents a word presented vocally by the examiner. "Lure" items are pictures that are phonemically similar to the target stimulus. The second and third parts of the battery are administered only if the child's performance on Part I is completed adequately. A training period precedes that actual test administration to familiarize the child with the vocabulary needed for the test. Summary scores are derived for each section; however, items are clustered into categories of specific sound contrasts through an item analysis. Thus, it is possible to obtain information regarding the specific speech-sound contrasts that are difficult for the child to perceive.

Goldman–Fristoe–Woodcock Tests of Auditory Selective Attention

The GFW Selective Attention Test (Goldman, Fristoe, & Woodcock, 1974–1976) consists of a variety of measures that assess auditory processing under varying conditions of background interference. Performance of the child is assessed under background conditions including a fan-like noise, a voice reading a story, and an ambient level of "cafeteria" noise. The response procedure is the same as that for the GFW tests noted above except that the target stimuli are given by prerecorded tape. Separate scores are derived for each of the three listening conditions. This set of tests requires 30–45 minutes for administration and a quiet (preferably sound-proof) room in which to give the test. Valuable information concerning the presence of a possible deficit in auditory figure-ground perception can be gathered from the Selective Attention subtest. Such information can be useful in educational treatment planning.

TACTILE FUNCTIONS

Reitan-Klove Sensory Perceptual Examination

This test assesses a variety of tactile, auditory, and visual perceptual functions and is relatively easy for the experienced clinician to administer. There are two forms of the test for children. The version of the test for older children, ages 9–15, is essentially the same as that used for adults and is discussed at length elsewhere (see Berg, Franzen, & Wedding, 1987). The second version of the test for children, ages 5–8 years, is a simplified version of the Reitan adult battery downward extension that was developed in 1955 as part of an overall downward extension of the adult battery (see Figure 10-4).

Originally, the sensory perceptual examination was developed by Reitan and Klove (Reitan, undated) based on similar tests used in neurology. The first part of the test evaluates the presence of sensory suppressions, using double simultaneous stimulation in the tactile, auditory, and visual modalities. Tests for perception of single stimulation are included since suppressions cannot be scored unless it is clear that the child is able to perceive unilateral stimulation. The child is asked to close her eyes and place her hand on the table. The examiner then proceeds randomly to touch either one of the child's hands, either side of her face, both hands, both sides of the face, or one hand and the opposite side of the face. *It is important that bilateral stimulation be done simultaneously and with equal pressure or else the child will be receiving two unilateral stimulations, thus defeating the purpose of the examination.* There should be no discernible pattern to the touching, and each hand as well as each side of the face should receive an equal number of both unilateral and simultaneous stimulations. The test is scored in terms of number of errors.

The presence of auditory perception deficits are assessed with the clinician standing behind the child and rubbing his fingers together slightly

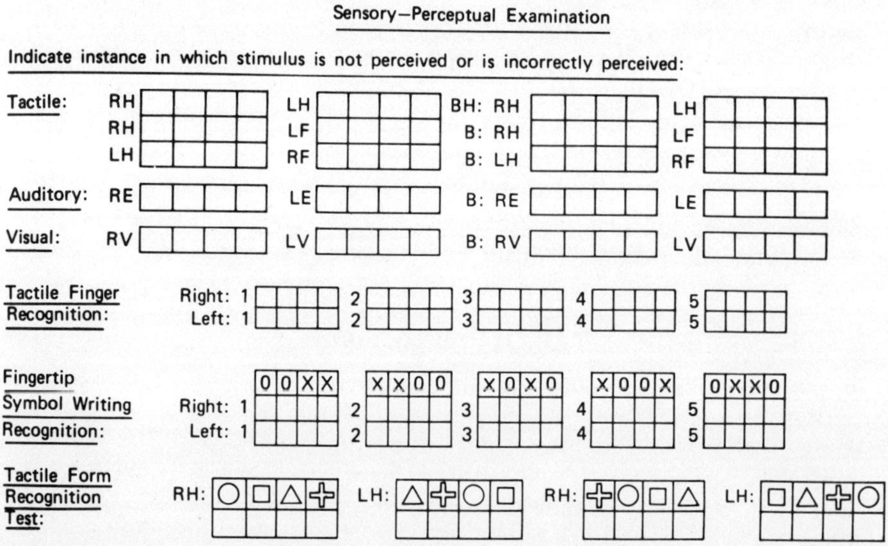
Sensory–Perceptual Examination

Indicate instance in which stimulus is not perceived or is incorrectly perceived:

Tactile: RH RH LH | LH LF RF | BH: RH B: RH B: LH | LH LF RF

Auditory: RE | LE | B: RE | LE

Visual: RV | LV | B: RV | LV

Tactile Finger Recognition: Right: 1 2 3 4 5; Left: 1 2 3 4 5

Fingertip Symbol Writing Recognition: O O X X | X X O O | X O X O | X O O X | O X X O; Right: 1 2 3 4 5; Left: 1 2 3 4 5

Tactile Form Recognition Test: RH: ○ □ △ ✚ | LH: △ ✚ ○ □ | RH: ✚ ○ □ △ | LH: □ △ ✚ ○

FIGURE 10-4. Sample of the Sensory Perceptual Examination Form for Young Children.

Screening Tests of Perceptual, Cognitive, and Motor Functioning 123

behind, but close to, the child's ears. The clinician then asks the child to tell on which side the noise was made—right, left, or both at once. The noise should be just audible to the child, and unilateral as well as bilateral simultaneous perceptual functioning should be assessed. As described above, total errors are scored.

Assessment for visual suppression is done in a similar manner. The examiner sits about three feet away from the front of the child and asks the child to fixate on the examiner's nose. The examiner's hands are then held at about an arm's length away from the examiner's body, and one or two fingers are moved slightly. The child is then asked on which side the movement occurred—left or right. Bilateral presentations also occur. An equal number of unilateral and double simultaneous stimulations should be given.

For all of the above, it is a good idea to practice with the child before actually starting the formal assessment to determine if the child is able to accurately distinguish left from right. If the child is consistently unable to identify the right or left side, the clinician can number the hands or use some other naming system. The child can also verbally respond by saying "Hand and face." Alternatively, the child may be instructed to raise the hand(s) and/or point to the appropriate side on which the stimulation was felt; however, this response form changes both the test and what is assessed somewhat, and the results will have to be interpreted cautiously. For the tactile and auditory portions of the test, the clinician may find that the child is unable to keep her eyes closed for an extended period of time. Use of a blindfold is an acceptable means of eliminating this problem. For the visual section of the test, the clinician must be extremely vigilant to ensure that the child is fixating in the center of the visual field and the child may have to be frequently prompted to maintain this fixation.

If no primary sensory deficit is in evidence, as indicated by correct identification of unilateral stimulations, even one error in double simultaneous stimulation can be indicative of cerebral dysfunction. The clinician must, however, be absolutely certain that the suppression error was a valid suppression and not the result of inattention. This is particularly true for children. *Genuine suppressions are quite rare but are almost always associated with brain injury.*

The Sensory Perceptual Examination for young children also contains a set of tests of more complex tactile perceptual functioning. The *Tactile Finger Recognition* test evaluates the child's ability to recognize which finger is touched while blindfolded (or with eyes closed). For this test, each finger is touched in random sequence by the examiner with the child telling the examiner which finger was touched. Some type of finger identification system that the child can understand and remember should be devised before the test actually begins. It is a good idea to practice with the child extensively before the beginning of the test. Generally, a simple numbering system, with the thumb being finger number one and the little finger being number five, works well, although if the child already has a naming system for her fingers, it is best to use that. In a similar manner, the Fingertip Symbol Writing Recognition test examines the blindfolded child's ability to recognize the symbols (x's and o's) written on the fingertips.

The Tactile Form Recognition test assesses for the presence of astereognosis. It involves the recognition of simple geometric shapes—a circle, square, triangle, Greek cross—by this touch. For this test, the child is instructed to place her right hand in a shadow box, and one of the shapes is placed in the hand. The child is then required to identify that shape that was placed in her hand by *pointing* to the correct shape in an array of shapes in front of her. The task is then repeated with the left hand, using the shapes in a different sequence. Both trials are then repeated, each time using a different sequence of shapes. For children, the test is scored for accuracy in shape identification only. Although normative data for this test are sparse, the normal child should make very few errors.

GENERAL COGNITIVE FUNCTIONS

The Stroop Test

The Stroop Test (Stroop, 1935) can be used as a measure of general cognitive efficiency in children as well as a measure of verbal fluency. In essence the Stroop assesses the ease with which the child is able to shift her perceptual set to conform to changing task demands. The most commonly used version of the Stroop was developed by Golden (1975). It consists of three $8\frac{1}{2}$ by 11-inch pages. Each item on the first page is one of the following words: red, green, or blue. These words are repeated on the page in a largely random order. The second page consists of 100 items, as does page 1, but each item is the sequence XXXX. On this page, each XXXX is printed in red, green, or blue ink. The third page consists of the words printed on page 1 in the colors used on page 2; however, a word and the color in which it is printed do not match. Therefore, "red" can be printed in either blue or green ink, "green" in red or blue ink, and "blue" in red or green ink.

The instructions for page 1 require that the child read down each column as quickly as possible, pronouncing the words printed. For page 2, the instructions are basically the same, except that the child is told to name the color of the XXXX. Finally, on the third page, the child is told to name the color of the ink rather than the word itself. Forty-five seconds are allotted for each page. These scores are then converted into standardized T-scores using tables in the test manual.

Golden (1979) has found that the Stroop is useful in the identification of dyslexia. Equivalent scores on pages 2 and 3 of the test are never seen in literate individuals. Thus, if the page 3 score is within 10–15% of the page-2 score, there is high likelihood of dyslexia, as this implies that the normal interference problem (words interfacing with color naming) has not occurred and that there is a dysfunction of word-reading skills.

Category Test

There are two versions of the Category Test for children. Both children's versions of the test are based on the adult version of the Category Test originally developed by Halstead (1947). In its original form, the adult version of the test was designed to assess abstraction. Stimulus figures, which vary in shape, size, number, intensity, color, and location and are grouped together by abstract principles, are projected on a screen. The individual must figure out the principle relating the stimulus subsets and respond by pressing the appropriate key on a simple keyboard. Correct responses are indicated by a bell that sounds automatically, whereas incorrect responses result in a harsh buzz. The adult version of the test consists of 208 items divided into seven subsets. The patient is told only that each subtest contains a single principle. Correct responses to the first few items are generally a matter of luck; however, she should quickly learn the pattern of bells and buzzes, and modify responding by developing and testing new hypotheses until the correct principle underlying the subtest is discerned. The patient is told at the end of each subset that a new subset is about to begin in which the underlying principle may be the same or different from the last subset.

Subset one requires the identification of eight Roman numerals. Subset two consists of 20 items, requiring the patient to respond to the number of items on the screen. The third section of the test contains 40 items and asks the individual to identify the position of the figure that is different from the others. Subtest four, also 40 items, requires that the patient determine one of the four quadrants of the figure that either has a missing part or is itself missing. Subset 5 contains 40 items, as does section six. Both portions of the test use the same underlying principle in which the salient characteristic of each stimulus is the proportion of the figure drawn with solid versus dashed lines (e.g., one quarter of the figure having solid lines requires a response of 1). The final subset (number 7) contains 20 items, some of which have already been seen by the patient during the test. The patient is told that it is necessary to remember and use the principles already used to get the correct response. For items not already used, the patient must determine the correct response in ways not totally dependent on recall of the previous subset items.

In the Category Test designed for children *ages 9 through 14* years, there are a total of 168 items distributed into six subsets (Reitan and Davison, 1974). The administration procedure is essentially the same as that for the adult version of the test. Some items from the adult test were reordered to attain a more consistent increase in level of difficulty, and all colored items were omitted. The 40-item fourth subset of the adult version was also eliminated. Finally, the summary sixth subtest consists only of those items that have actually appeared before as claimed in the instructions (Boll, 1981). The test was designed to assess concept formation in children as well as mental efficiency, and to some extent, learning skills (Teeter, 1986). The test is sensitive to global or a generalized dysfunction.

The version of the Category Test designed for young children *ages 5 through 8* was again changed to simplify the response pattern required from the child (Reitan, 1969). Boll (1981) noted that it would be incorrect to assume that children in this age range are all familiar with numbers, particularly those in the lower portion of the age distribution. For this reason, the lights over the response levers on the keyboard were changed from the numbers 1, 2, 3, and 4 to colors (red, blue, yellow, and green). The stimulus characteristics of the colors were designed to minimize, if not eliminate, potential disadvantages due to color blindness. This version of the test was shortened to 80 items in five subsets. Color knowledge of naming is also not required. Rather, some aspect of the stimulus was designed to suggest a particular color, and if the response lever under that color is pulled, the child is reinforced with the bell. An incorrect response results in the buzzer.

The first subset of 10 items requires that the child choose the response lever under the color that appears on the screen. The next three subtests—2, 3, and 4—have 20 items each. Subset 2 requires a response based on the color that is present on the screen in the greatest quantity for each item. For subtest 2, an "oddity" principle is used; some characteristic of the stimulus other than color (size, shape) determines the correct response. In subtest 4, the child must determine the color which either is absent or least predominating on the screen for each item. In the final subtest, the child is asked to recall the correct principle from previously seen items for each of the 10 items in the subset.

Wisconsin Card Sorting Test

The Wisconsin Card Sorting Test (WCST) was devised to study "abstract behavior" and the ability to "shift set" (Berg, 1948; Grant & Berg, 1948). The child is given a pack of 64 cards on which are printed one to four symbols—star, cross, circle, or triangle—in green, red, yellow, or blue. No two cards are identical. The child is asked to place them one by one under four stimulus cards—one red triangle, two green stars, three yellow crosses, and four blue circles—according to a principle that she must deduce from

Screening Tests of Perceptual, Cognitive, and Motor Functioning

the pattern of the clinician's responses to the child's placement of the cards. For example, if the principle is color, the correct placement of a blue card is under the four circles, regardless of the symbol or number, and the examiner responds accordingly. After 10 consecutive correct placements, the examiner changes the principle being used for placement, indicating the change only in the altered pattern of the "right" and "wrong" statements given to the child. The test begins with color as the first principle, changes to form, then to number, returns to color again, and so on. The test continues until the child has made six runs of two correct placements, has placed more than 64 cards in one category, or uses 128 cards (Heaton, 1981).

A variety of cognitive deficits can lead to poor performance. The child may have difficulty in sorting according to category, suggesting problems in forming abstract concepts. Perseveration (difficulty in shifting the principle used) is another common error. Chelune and Baer (1986) have developed normative data for children as young as 6 years of age. In addition, they have found that from about age 10 and up, normal performance for a child is essentially the same as that seen in the adult normative data gathered by Heaton (1981) (see Table 10-5).

Porteus Mazes

Maze tracing tasks were originally designed to yield data about the highest levels of cognitive functioning involving planning and foresight (Lezak, 1983). Porteus (1959, p. 7) noted that the test evaluates, in some measure, "the process of choosing, trying, and rejecting or adopting alternative courses or thought. At a simple level, this is similar to solving a very complex maze." Maze tests are useful in measuring general ability as well as specific nonverbal reasoning and visuopractic functions (Lezak, 1983).

There are currently three versions of the Porteus Mazes in use. The Vinland Revision contains 12 mazes for years III through XII, year XIV, and

TABLE 10-5 Normal WCST Performance

		Age							
		6	7	8	9	10	11	12	Adult
Categories	M	2.73	4.07	4.05	4.81	5.60	5.58	5.70	5.40
Achieved	SD	2.10	1.94	2.01	1.47	0.75	0.79	0.95	1.30
Perseverative	M	40.64	25.07	23.18	18.13	13.95	15.17	12.30	12.60
Errors	SD	28.03	18.43	13.23	11.55	6.50	13.49	16.94	10.20
Failures to	M	1.64	1.93	1.82	1.75	1.00	1.17	0.70	0.80
Maintain Set	SD	2.01	1.21	1.26	1.53	1.02	1.11	0.68	1.30

Adapted from Chelune, G. J., & Baer, R. A. 1986). Developmental norms for the Wisconsin card sorting test. *Journal of Clinical and Experimental Neuropsychology, 8,* 219–228. Adapted with permission.

Adult. The Porteus Maze Extension consists of eight mazes that are used for years VII through XII, year XIV, and Adult. There is also the Porteus Maze Supplement which has eight mazes for years VII through XII, XIV, and Adult (Porteus, 1965) (see Figure 10-5). The latter two series of mazes were developed to allow for practice effects seen in retesting. The maze at each year of the Porteus Maze Extension is a little more difficult than its counterpart in the Vineland Revision, and each year of the Porteus Maze Supplement is somewhat more difficult than its counterpart in the Extension mazes (Lezak, 1983).

To complete a trial successfully, the child must trace the maze without entering any blind alleys. If a blind alley is entered, the maze is immediately removed from the child and another copy of the same maze is placed in front of her and the child is instructed to attempt the maze a second time. Each maze has a specified number of trials that can be attempted before a failure is recorded. The test is not timed and, because of this, can take a good deal of time for the child to complete all mazes given to her. Scores are

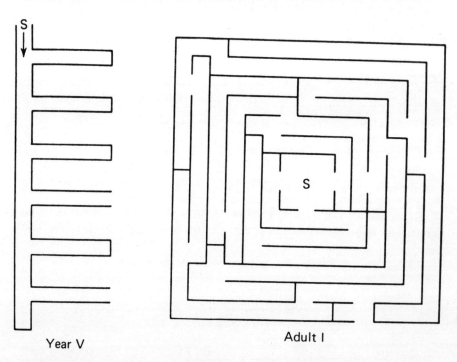

FIGURE 10-5. Two of the Porteus Mazes.

Reproduced by permission. Copyright © 1933, 1946, 1950 by S. D. Porteus. Published by the Psychological Corporation, San Antonio, Texas. All rights reserved.

reported in terms of test age, and a qualitative scoring system also is available with the test.

The Porteus Maze Test has been found to be quite sensitive to the effects of general brain injury in both children and adults (Smith, 1960; Smith and Kinder, 1959).

WISC-R Mazes Subtest

The Wechsler Intelligence Scale for Children-Revised (WISC-R; Wechsler, 1974) contains a maze subtest that is shorter that the Porteus Mazes with time limits and an error scoring system. It consists of nine printed mazes of varying sizes and complexity which are administered in order of difficulty. Scoring is based on the number of errors with standard scores derived from the age-appropriate normative data table.

MANUAL MOTOR FUNCTIONING

Generally, it is a good idea to include a measure or measures of manual motor control and speed in a screening battery. All such tests are timed speed tests that either have an apparatus with a counting device or require a countable response from the child. Such tests have been useful in the detection of lateralized brain dysfunction.

Finger Tapping Test

Perhaps the most widely used test of motor functioning is the Finger Tapping Test (Reitan & Davison, 1974), which was originally called the Finger Oscillation Test by Halstead (1947). It consists of a tapping key with a device for recording the number of taps. Each hand performs three 10-second trials with brief rest period interspersed between trials. The score for each hand is then averaged across the three trials. Normal performance varies with age (see Table 10-4). The presence of cortical damage tends to have a slowing effect on the rate of finger tapping. Lateralized lesions may result in a marked slowing of the tapping rate of the hand contralateral to the lesion. However, such effects do not appear with enough frequency or consistency to warrant the use of this test as a screening for lateralized damage. Diffuse damage will lead to a generalized slowing of the tapping rate of both hands. In general, there is roughly a 10% difference in the tapping rates of the two hands, with the dominant hand being faster.

When the children's version of the test was first devised, an electronic tapper was introduced to present a task that was easier for children who

TABLE 10-4 Finger Tapping Test Scores for Normal Control Subjects

		Age									
		5	6	7	8	9	10	11	12	13	14
Dominant hand	M	24.31	28.15	29.78	33.75	33.90	37.37	40.90	41.61	45.97	46.32
	SD	4.83	3.48	4.72	5.09	4.12	5.43	4.79	4.89	5.80	6.04
Nondominant hand	M	22.14	25.36	26.82	29.86	30.20	33.28	36.48	36.89	42.01	42.18
	SD	4.21	3.01	4.17	4.71	3.27	4.86	4.75	3.88	4.58	5.45

Adapted from Klonoff, H. & Low, M. (1976). Disordered brain function in young children and early adolescents: Neuropsychological and electroencephalographic correlates. In R. M. Reitan and L. A. Davison (Eds.), *Clinical neuropsychology: Current status and applications* (pp. 121–178), Washington, D.C.; V. H. Winston & Sons. Adapted with permission.

Screening Tests of Perceptual, Cognitive, and Motor Functioning

have shorter fingers than adults. The technical disadvantages of the procedure, however, were found to outweigh the advantages. Young children are able to manage well with the manual tapper and using the electronic tapper is not truly necessary (Boll, 1981).

Grip Strength

Examining the child's level of performance and comparing performance on both sides of the body can be useful in determining the integrity of brain functioning. Clinicians have realized that intensity or strength of voluntary motor activity also can be a reliable indicator of brain functioning. Many neuropsychologists use some strength-of-grip measure in comprehensive evaluations. Such a measure is also appropriate as a part of a general screening of brain function.

Reitan and Davison (1974) established the hand dynamometer as having clinical value for such purposes. Testing the strength of a child's grip requires the use of a dynamometer which can be adjusted to the size of the child's hand. The child is asked to extend her preferred hand downward and is then instructed to squeeze as hard as possible. Two trials are given to each hand in alternating sequence. The two trials for each hand should be within three to five kilograms of each other. The final score for each hand is the average of the two trials. The child's performance is then compared with appropriate normative data (see Table 10-5).

Clinicians who may be interested in using the Grip Strength test should be warned that although the test is a reasonably good indicator of brain dysfunction in a number of instances, it cannot be used as the sole measure; it is not accurate enough to do so. In addition, hand dynamometers are not inexpensive. The current cost of a hand dynamometer ranges from $175 to $275 depending on the brand and supplier.

Purdue Pegboard

The Purdue Pegboard (Purdue Research Foundation, 1948) is a sensory-motor test that has been used as a screening device for the detection of neurological dysfunction both in adults and school-age children (Costa, Vaughan, Levit, & Farber, 1963; Rapin, Tourk, & Costa, 1966). Normative data have recently been made available for young children aged 2 years, 6 months through 5 years, 11 months (see Table 10-6; Wilson, Iacoviello, Wilson, & Risucci, 1982). Following standardized instructions for individuals aged 6 and up, the child places pegs in holes with her left hand, right hand, and then both hands simultaneously. Each trial lasts for 30 seconds, so that the total actual testing time is only 90 seconds. The score is

TABLE 10-6 Purdue Pegboard Normative Data for Preschool-Age Children

Age interval (years and months)	Right hand		Left hand		Both hands	
	M	SD	M	SD	M	SD
2–6 to 2–11	4.70	1.08	4.05	1.15	2.95	1.28
3–0 to 3–5	5.54	1.62	5.13	1.42	3.63	1.53
3–6 to 3–11	6.80	1.26	6.00	1.38	4.20	1.23
4–0 to 4–5	8.08	1.49	6.68	1.25	5.23	1.44
4–6 to 4–11	9.07	1.58	8.20	1.56	6.07	1.20
5–0 to 5–5	10.16	1.77	9.19	2.02	6.81	1.76
5–6 to 5–11	9.90	1.59	9.00	1.26	6.35	1.69

Mean score is the mean number of pegs for each hand. For the "Both Hands" condition, the score is the mean number of pairs of pegs placed.

Adapted from Wilson, B. C., Iacoviello, J. M., Wilson, J. J., & Risucci, D. (1982). Purdue Pegboard performance of normal preschool children. *Journal of Clinical Neuropsychology, 4,* 19–26. Adapted with permission.

the number of pegs placed correctly. Normative data are available for the test although cutting scores can be used.

For the younger children's version, the pegboard has been cut down to accommodate the shorter reach of younger children. Separate scores are available for preferred and nonpreferred hands individually as well as for both hands working simultaneously.

In general, for individuals of all ages, a brain lesion is likely to be present whenever the score of the nonpreferred hand exceeds that of the preferred hand, or the score of the preferred hand exceeds that of the nonpreferred hand by three or more points. Slowing on one hand is suggestive of a dysfunction in the contralateral hemisphere, and bilateral slowing typically occurs with diffuse or bilateral brain damage.

Since the total testing time, including instructions and practice, rarely exceeds 5 minutes, the Purdue Pegboard test can be a highly efficient method of screening for cortical dysfunction and detecting a lateralized lesion. Since it is not only brief but also unlikely to fatigue a child unduly, it can be included in most neuropsychological test screening batteries. The test's size and weight may place limits on its portability in some situations, however.

11
Verbal Screening Instruments

Verbal communication is, perhaps, one of the most important aspects of a child's total development. Learning to communicate adequately is virtually essential for survival in our verbal world. A child should have intact and functional speech, language, and hearing abilities. Deficits in any one, or combination, of these areas can contribute to a basic communication disorder and potentially have an untoward impact on the child's ability for independent survival. Speech, language, and hearing skills are fundamental functions in the overall learning process.

A variety of professional disciplines have contributed to a more comprehensive understanding of verbally related disorders. These disciplines include audiology, speech pathology, and neuropsychology, to name a few. Clearly, a comprehensive discussion of each of these specialties and its relative contribution to understanding communication is well beyond the scope of this chapter. Along the same lines, the clinician interested in screening for the presence of a brain-based disorder is not going to perform a comprehensive speech and language evaluation, nor is he going to conduct an audiological evaluation. Rather, the general clinician working with children will be interested in attempting to determine the possible presence of a language disorder and will likely then make the appropriate referral for an in-depth evaluation.

This chapter, therefore, will be limited to a discussion of some of the commonly available, and easily and rapidly administered assessment devices and techniques that can be used to make an initial determination of verbal functioning in children. In addition, we will attempt to present a brief chronology of "normal" language development to assist the clinician in recognizing possible abnormal language development.

"NORMAL" LANGUAGE DEVELOPMENT

A child's language acquisition tends to be hierarchical and follows a regular schedule to some extent. What follows is a representation of the normal language learning "schedule" in children based on the work of Bartel (1975), Menyuk (1971), and Byrne and Shervanian (1977). The clinician must remember that there is a tremendous amount of individual difference among children and that the information presented here is not only idealized to some degree, but also is a distillation of a large literature on the subject.

From birth through 6 months of age, the infant will begin to produce vocalizations such as coos, cries, grunts, and gasps. Between the ages of 6 and 9 months, the infant's vocabulary is essentially jargon that is characterized by some syllables being present as is intonation. Typically, the infant responds to speech by smiling and by producing various vocalizations that are acoustically similar to adult utterances and that will vary from one situation to another. At 9 months of age, the infant enters the jargon stage of speech in which an identifiable stress and intonation pattern begins to emerge as does some imitation of language-like patterns. During the babbling stage, ages 9–12 months, the infant's "language" is characterized by a type of echolalia in which sounds made by the infant and others are repeated. It is in this stage that the first words are often uttered. The infant will have some receptive ability and will perform meaningful language-based behaviors such as wave "bye-bye."

In the next six months (12–18 months of age), the beginnings of true intentionally used speech are usually seen. The child will develop a 1–20 word vocabulary and generally will respond to simple commands and one-word phrases. The mean utterance during this period is one word. From 18 to 24 months of age, meaningful speech is developed and the child has a vocabulary of up to about 300 words. He will produce two-word sentences, and single words are often used to represent entire phrases. Comprehension usually exceeds verbal production. In other words, the child is able to understand much of what is said to him during the second year of life.

Between the ages of 2 and 3 years, the child's speech becomes more intelligible as he begins to acquire some of the more common grammatical rules. Normal speech dysfluencies begin to disappear. The child's vocabulary increases to 900 or more words. The average utterance is 3 to 4 words and he begins to comprehend grammatical tense and basic number concepts but is not yet able to produce them consistently. During the next year (ages 3–4), language increases in its complexity and becomes more refined with a concomitant increase in the use of various parts of speech. The average utterance is now four to eight words and the child is able to comprehend most adult language structure as well as more number concepts. The child's vocabulary increases to about 1500 words during this year.

From ages 4 to 5, the child's vocabulary expands to upwards of 2,500 words and he typically says seven or more words at a time. The child's language becomes more abstract in nature, and there is more language form and structure to the child's speech. Knowledge of opposites begins to occur as does the use of "how" and "why" questions. The child is also beginning to be able to define specific words at this time. Generally, between 3 and 5 years of age the child employs a more varied sentence structure that although functionally complete, is grammatically incomplete. Sentence structure ranges from simple to compound and complex.

At 5 to 6 years of age, language continues to be refined, vocabulary is well above 2,500 words, and the average sentence length is 4.5 words. Analysis of speech at this time reveals an inner logic to the speech as well as some abstraction and categorization. Language becomes more symbolic between the ages of 6 and 7. "Serious" reading and writing are also started. The child's speech is characterized by words that are increased in both size and complexity. The child is now better able to define terms, offer meaningful explanations, has developed an understanding of time and the seasons, and is also starting to be able to correctly identify right and left. By the age of 7, the average child is able to use language fluently; in fact, he likes to use bigger and more complex words. The child also begins to demonstrate that he comprehends cause-and-effect relationships. From this point onward, the child's language will continue to develop depending on native ability, and environmental opportunity.

LANGUAGE DISORDERS IN CHILDREN

Disruptions of language functioning may come to the attention of the clinician in a variety of forms. For instance, a child may demonstrate a significant delay in beginning to speak or may exhibit a persistent difficulty in comprehending speech. One of the first things the clinician may be called on to do is to determine whether the problem represents a failure or delay in acquiring language, or a complete loss or reduction in the child's language capacity that has occurred subsequent to language acquisition (Spreen, Tupper, Risser, Tuokko, & Edgell, 1984).

Marge (1972) has defined three basic categories into which the distinction must be made: (1) the failure to acquire language (children who are 4 years of age have not shown any sign of acquiring language); (2) delayed language acquisition (children whose language level is below that of their age peers); and (3) an acquired language disorder (children who at some

TABLE 11-1 Differential Diagnosis of Language Disorders in Childhood

Hearing loss
Oral-area sensory deficits
Aphasia
    Acquired
    Congenital
    Developmental
Dyslexia
    Acquired
    Developmental
Minimal brain dysfunction
Childhood psychosis
Nonpsychotic functional behavior disorders
Epilepsy
Mental retardation
Environmental deficits (sensory, emotional, cultural deprivation, inadequate or incomplete academic instruction)
Normal variation

From Spreen, O. S., Tupper, D., Risser, A., Tuokko, H., & Edgell, D. (1984). *Human Developmental Neuropsychology,* New York: Oxford University Press. Reprinted by permission of Oxford University Press.

point in development acquired language and who subsequently suffered a complete loss or a reduction in their capacity to use language). Table 11-1 presents the differential diagnoses of language disorders with which the clinician may be faced.

There are a number of considerations that can help the clinician clarify the nature of language disorders and aid in the differential diagnosis. If the disorder occurs in the absence of intellectual deficit and serious environmental deprivation, it is generally referred to as either *dysphasia* or aphasia, although Spreen et al (1984) note that dysphasia remains the term of preference for congenital disorders. Frequently, the language disorder will occur in the context of other, more pervasive disorders such as deafness, mental retardation, and severe childhood psychiatric disorders. Depending on the nature of the clinician's practice, he may be called on to make such a differential diagnosis.

CHILDHOOD APHASIA

Although acquired language disorders probably represent the smallest proportion of children affected with language disorders, the study of these children has yielded the most striking evidence about the complexities inherent in the study of the developing central nervous sytem. The effects during infancy and childhood of acquired brain injuries on language functioning differ markedly from the effects of lesions acquired by adults. For example, one noteworthy feature of childhood aphasia, in contrast to adult aphasia, is the reduction in the amount of speech produced regardless of the location of the lesion (Alajouanine & Lhermitte, 1965; Guttman, 1942; Karlin, 1954; Rapin, Mattis, Rowan, & Golden, 1977).

It has been reported that the aphasic child may not only demonstrate reduced verbal output, but also may be reluctant to communicate or exchange information through other modalities such as writing or using gestures (Alajouanine & Lhermitte, 1965; Karlin, 1954). In adults, a dominant hemisphere injury typically leads to language disorders whereas in children, large brain lesions sustained early in life, even if treated by the removal of an entire hemisphere, do not produce profound language impairment, regardless of the side of the brain involved. Such research and clinical findings and the observation that children recover language functions more rapidly than adults have been one major basis for theories about the ontogeny of cerebral dominance and plasticity, and critical periods for development of functional capabilities.

Reviews of the literature on childhood acquired aphasia confirmed earlier suggestions for an initial hemispheric equipotentiality for language (Dennis & Whitaker, 1977; Satz & Bullard-Bates, 1981). This assumption appears to hold up approximately to the age of 1 year. Whereas prior to this age, a right-sided hemiplegia produces a one-to-one risk for language impairment, the frequency of aphasia associated with right hemiplegia increases dramatically after this age, and by the age of 5 years, it approximates the ratios found in adults.

These findings, however, are somewhat modified by the studies of hemispherectomy reviewed by Ludlow (1979). Ludlow's report suggests that although phonemic discrimination and lexicon may have an equal potential in the right and left hemisphere, the discrimination of complex syntactic material may be more seriously impaired by left hemispherectomy. This seems to suggest that the left hemisphere may be responsible for a nonredundant (in the right hemisphere) language behavior, that being syntactic complexity (Ludlow, 1979). Dennis (1980), in a review of hemispherectomy studies, stresses that the left hemisphere also "allows for the development of a set of semantic abilities not available to the right" (p, 183).

As is the case with adults, almost any verbal test can be considered a test for aphasia, since children with language disorder tend to do more poorly than do children without such disorders. Specific tests for aphasia, however, differ from other verbal assessment instruments in that they have been designed to focus on disorders of symbol formulation as well as associated agnosias and apraxias (Benton, 1967). These tests operate by eliciting samples of a child's behavior in various communication/language modalities of listening, reading, writing, and gesturing. The clinician must select a testing device that can sample all such language-related behaviors quickly and efficiently.

An aphasia screening test is not designed to replace the careful examination of language functions afforded by comprehensive language assessment batteries; however, such a test can signal the presence of a disorder and may even call attention to its specific characteristics. It does not provide the fine discriminations of the more complete aphasia test batteries (Eisensen, 1973). Since these tests do not require technical knowledge of speech pathology for satisfactory administration or interpretation, they can be easily administered and interpreted by clinicians who are not necessarily familiar with the various syndromes of aphasia.

TESTS FOR APHASIA

Aphasia Screening Test

Since its introduction, this has become perhaps one of most widely used of all aphasia tests. The Aphasia Screening Test (AST) or one of its many variations has been incorporated into many formally organized neuropsychological test batteries. As originally devised by Halstead and Wepman (1959), the AST has 51 items that cover all the elements of aphasic disabilities as well as the most common language problems. The total time for administration rarely is more than 30 minutes and is often far shorter. There are no rigid scoring standards for the AST since the emphasis is placed on determining both the presence, and to a lesser extent, the nature, of communication problems. Errors are coded into a diagnostic profile that provides a description of the individual's language deficits. The test is not designed to assess performance on the basis of serverity of the problem; however, the more areas of involvement noted, the greater the likelihood of a more severe dysfunction.

Reitan included the AST with a number of other different tests in the Halstead–Reitan Neuropsychological Battery, which is described in detail elsewhere (e.g., see Reitan & Davison, 1974). He reduced the original test to 32 items, but still handled data in a descriptive fashion in much the same manner as originally intended. This shortened version of the AST is one of the most commonly used and is readily available for both adults and older children, ages 9–14. Table 11-2 and Figure 11-1 present the tasks in the AST as well as the organization of the items.

For younger children, ages 5 to 8 years, Reitan (1955) developed a shortened and simplified version of the AST. The test is reduced to 22 items which have been simplified to take into account normal expectations for children in this age range (see Table 11-3). The stimulus materials used for

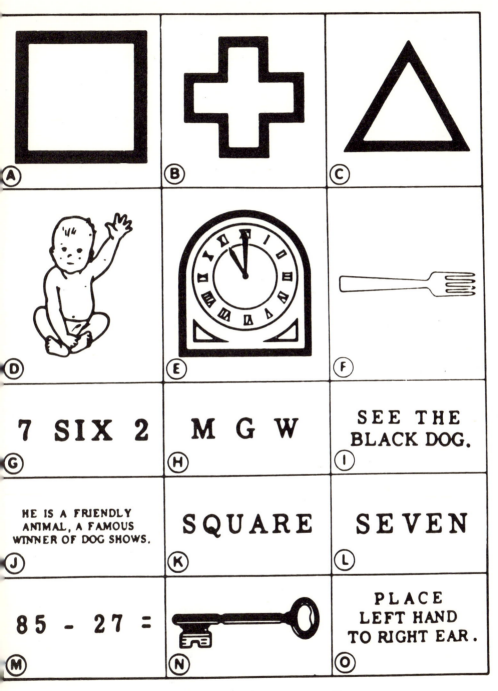

FIGURE 11-1. Stimulus figures for the Aphasia Screening Test.

From Boll, T. J. (1981). The Halstead-Reitan Neuropsychological Test Battery. In S. B. Filskov & T. J. Boll (Eds.), *Handbook of clinical neusopsychology.* New York: Wiley-Interscience. Copyright © 1981. Reprinted by permission of John Wiley & Sons, Inc.

TABLE 11-2 Aphasia Screening Test Items for Older Children (Ages 9–14)

Task	Instruction to child
1. Copy SQUARE (A)	FIRST, DRAW THIS ON PAPER. (Point to square, item A.) I WANT YOU TO DO IT WITHOUT LIFTING YOUR PENCIL FROM THE PAPER. TRY TO MAKE IT ABOUT THE SAME SIZE. (Elaborate as necessary.) If the child is concerned about making a heavy of double line, note that only a reproduction of the shape is necessary. If the child encounters difficulty in shape reproduction, encourage the child to do his or her best. If the task is not accomplished reasonably well on the first attempt, ask the child to try again.
2. Name SQUARE	WHAT IS THAT SHAPE CALLED?
3. Spell SQUARE	WOULD YOU SPELL THAT WORD FOR ME?
4. Copy CROSS (B)	DRAW THIS ON YOUR PAPER. (Point to cross.) GO AROUND THE OUTSIDE LIKE THIS UNTIL YOU GET BACK WHERE YOU STARTED. (Examiner draws a finger line around the edge of the figure.) MAKE IT ABOUT THE SAME SIZE. Additional instructions are given in the same manner as those used for the square as needed.
5. Name CROSS	WHAT IS THAT SHAPE CALLED?
6. Spell CROSS	WOULD YOU SPELL THAT WORD FOR ME?
7. Copy TRIANGLE (C)	Similar to instructions for 1 and 4.
8. Name TRIANGLE	WHAT IS THAT SHAPE CALLED?
9. Spell TRIANGLE	WOULD YOU SPELL THAT WORD FOR ME?
10. Name BABY (D)	WHAT IS THIS? (Show item D.)
11. Write CLOCK (E)	NOW I AM GOING TO SHOW YOU ANOTHER PICTURE BUT DO NOT TELL ME THE NAME OF IT. DON'T SAY ANYTHING OUT LOUD. JUST WRITE THE NAME OF THE PICTURE ON THE PAPER. (Show item E.)
12. Name FORK (F)	WHAT IS THIS? (Show item F.)
13. Read 7 SIX 2 (G)	I WANT YOU TO READ THIS. (Show item G.) If the child has difficulty, attempt to determine if any of the stimulus figure can be read.
14. Read M G W (H)	READ THIS. (Show item H.)
15. Reading I (I)	READ THIS. (Show item I.)
16. Reading II (J)	TRY TO READ THIS. (Show item J.)
17. Repeat TRIANGLE	NOW I AM GOING TO SAY SOME WORDS. I WANT YOU TO LISTEN CAREFULLY AND SAY THEM AS CAREFULLY AS YOU CAN. SAY THIS WORD: TRIANGLE.
18. Repeat MASSACHUSETTS	THE NEXT ONE IS A LITTLE HARDER BUT TRY TO DO YOUR BEST. SAY: MASSACHUSETTS
19. Repeat METHODIST EPISCOPAL	NOW REPEAT THIS ONE: METHODIST EPISCOPAL
20. Write SQUARE (K)	DON'T SAY THIS WORD OUT LOUD. (Point to item K.) JUST WRITE IT ON YOUR PAPER. If the child prints the words, ask him to write it in script or cursive, if he knows how.

Verbal Screening Instruments

TABLE 11-2 Continued

Task	Instruction to child
21. Read SEVEN (L).	READ THIS WORD OUT LOUD. (Show item L.)
22. Repeat SEVEN	NOW, I WANT YOU TO SAY THIS AFTER ME: SEVEN
23. Repeat and explain HE SHOUTED THE WARNING	I AM GOING TO SAY SOMETHING THAT I WANT YOU TO SAY AFTER ME. LISTEN CAREFULLY: HE SHOUTED THE WARNING. NOW YOU SAY IT. PLEASE EXPLAIN WHAT THAT SENTENCE MEANS. Sometimes the examiner will have to ask for additional explanations by asking the kind of situation to which the sentence refers. The child must indicate that danger is impending.
24. Write HE SHOUTED THE WARNING	NOW, WRITE THAT SENTENCE ON THE PAPER. The sentence can be repeated if necessary.
25. Compute $85 - 27 =$ (M)	HERE IS AN ARITHMETIC PROBLEM. COPY IT ON THE PAPER AND TRY TO SOLVE IT. (Show item M.)
26. Compute $17 \times 3 =$	NOW DO THIS ONE IN YOUR HEAD. HOW MUCH IS 17×3?
27. Name KEY (N)	WHAT IS THIS? (Show item N.)
28. Demonstrate use of KEY (N)	SHOW ME HOW TO USE THIS IF YOU HAD ONE IN YOUR HAND. (Show item N.)
29. Draw KEY (N)	NOW, PLEASE DRAW A PICTURE THAT LOOKS LIKE THIS ONE. TRY TO MAKE YOUR KEY LOOK ENOUGH LIKE THE ONE IN THE PICTURE SO THAT SOMEONE WOULD KNOW IT WAS THE SAME KEY IN THE DRAWING. (Point to item N.)
30. Read (O)	WOULD YOU READ THIS? (Show item O.)
31. Place LEFT HAND TO RIGHT EAR	PLEASE DO WHAT IT SAID.
32. Place LEFT HAND TO LEFT ELBOW	NOW I WANT YOU TO PUT YOUR LEFT HAND ON YOUR LEFT ELBOW. The child should realize that this is not possible.

Adapted from Boll, T. J. (1981). The Halstead–Reitan Neuropsychological Battery. In S. B. Filskov & T. J. Boll (Eds.), *Handbook of clinical neuropsychology.* New York: Wiley-Interscience. Copyright © 1981. Adapted by permission of John Wiley & Sons, Inc.

those items requiring such materials in the young children's version of the test are the same as those used with the version of the AST for older children and adults.

The Token Test

The Token Test is very easy to administer, easy to score, and generally easy for children to perform with few, if any, errors. It was originally introduced by DeRenzi and Vignolo (1962) as a sensitive measure to detect subtle receptive language deficits in aphasic adults. In the DeRenzi and Vignolo Token Test, as well as in several other forms of the test subsequently

TABLE 11-3 Aphasia Screening Test Items for Young Children (Ages 5–8)

Task	Instructions to child
1. Write NAME	I WANT YOU TO WRITE YOUR NAME ON THE PAPER IN FRONT OF YOU. IF YOU KNOW HOW TO WRITE YOUR LAST NAME, DO THAT TOO. If the child prints, ask if he knows how to write in cursive or script. If he does, ask him to write his name again in cursive. If he does not know how, printing is acceptable.
2. Copy SQUARE (A)	FIRST, DRAW THIS ON YOUR PAPER. (Point to square, item A.) I WANT YOU TO DO IT WITHOUT LIFTING YOUR PENCIL FROM THE PAPER. TRY TO MAKE IT ABOUT THE SAME SIZE. (Elaborate as necessary.) If the child is concerned about making a heavy of double line, note that only a reproduction of the shape is necessary. If the child encounters difficulty in shape reproduction, encourage the child to do his or her best. If the task is not accomplished reasonably well on the first attempt, ask the child to try again.
3. Copy CROSS (B)	DRAW THIS ON YOUR PAPER. (Point to cross.) GO AROUND THE OUTSIDE LIKE THIS UNTIL YOU GET BACK WHERE YOU STARTED. (Examiner draws a finger line around the edge of the figure.) MAKE IT ABOUT THE SAME SIZE. Additional instructions are given in the same manner as those used for the square as needed.
4. Copy TRIANGLE (C)	Similar to instructions for 2 and 3.
5. Name BABY (D)	WHAT IS THIS? (Show item D.)
6. Name CLOCK (E)	NOW I AM GOING TO SHOW YOU ANOTHER PICTURE. WHAT IS THIS? (Show item E.)
7. Name FORK (F)	WHAT IS THIS? (Show item F.)
8. Read 7 SIX 2 (G)	I WANT YOU TO READ THIS. (Show item G.) If the child has difficulty, attempt to determine if any of the stimulus figure can be read.
9. Read M G W (H)	READ THIS. (Show item H.)
10. Read SEE THE BLACK DOG	READ THIS. (Show item I.)
11. Print SQUARE (K)	DON'T SAY THIS WORD OUT LOUD (Point to item K.) JUST PRINT IT ON YOUR PAPER.
12. COUNT FINGERS	I WANT YOU TO COUNT THE FINGERS ON BOTH HANDS FOR ME. Indicate that the child is to start with the thumb of one hand and continue to the little finger before starting with the thumb of the other hand.
13. Compute 2 + 2 (Verbal)	TELL ME, HOW MUCH IS 2 + 2?
14. Compute 2 + 1 (Written)	HERE IS AN ARITHMETIC PROBLEM. The examiner writes the problem on the paper: $\begin{array}{r}2\\+1\\\hline\end{array}$ or $2 + 1 =$ TRY TO SOLVE IT.

TABLE 11-3 Continued

Task	Instructions to child
15. Compute 4 + 3 (Verbal)	NOW DO THIS ONE IN YOUR HEAD. HOW MUCH IS 4 + 3?
16. Name KEY (N)	WHAT IS THIS? (Show item N.)
17. Put FINGER ON NOSE	I WOULD LIKE YOU TO PUT YOUR FINGER ON YOUR NOSE. The child may use either hand.
18. Show TONGUE	SHOW ME YOUR TONGUE. The child may either point to his tongue or stick his tongue out at the examiner.
19. Where is EYEBROW?	WHERE IS YOUR EYEBROW? SHOW ME or POINT TO IT. The child must either point to or touch the eyebrow. The eyelid is not acceptable. If unsure of where the child is pointing, ask the child to touch the eyebrow.
20. Point to ELBOW	Instructions are similar to item 19.
21. Put RIGHT HAND on NOSE	PUT YOUR RIGHT HAND ON YOUR NOSE.
22. Put LEFT HAND on HEAD	PUT YOUR LEFT HAND ON YOUR HEAD.

devised by other researchers, the patient is asked to manipulate different colored and shaped objects. Despite all the various changes in the test that have been made by various investigators, the Token Test remains remarkably sensitive to disrupted linguistic processes that are central to aphasic disorders, even when the patient's basic ability to communiate has remained intact (e.g., Spreen & Benton, 1969; Wilson, 1986). The test can also identify those brain-damaged individuals whose other disabilities may be hiding or masking a concomitant aphasic disorder, or whose problems with symbol processing are comparatively subtle and not readily observable in the majority of situations. The test was originally designed to meet a number of ideal conditions for language tests that include sampling linguistic, but not intellectual abilities, sampling various levels of linguistic difficulty without the use of obscure language, sampling language without the use of extensive memorization, and sampling language within a relatively brief period of time.

More recently, the test has been used to assess language function in children (Wilson, 1986). The test is comprised of 20 "tokens," usually cut from heavy construction paper, thin sheets of plastic, or wood. They come in two shapes—circles and squares (although rectangles can be used just as easily); two sizes—large and small; and five colors—blue, green, yellow, white, and red. The only requirement that the test makes of the child is that he understand the token names and the verbs and prepositions in the instructions. The child should be informally tested prior to the actual test administration to make sure he understands the meaning of the words *circle* and *square, large* and *small,* and can identify all five colors of the tokens. (Three- and four-year-old children may have some difficulty with these concepts. If this is the case, the test should be discontinued and alternative testing instruments be used.) The instructions are then read to the child *only once.* The test is divided into five parts, each of which presents progressively longer and more complex commands, for a total of 61 items (see Table 11-4). Although the Token Test seems easy to administer, the clinician must be careful not to modify the rate of delivery inadvertently in response to the quality of the child's performance. In addition, all test commands should be spoken clearly with *no emphasis or stress on any words.* If the child asks to have an item repeated, the examiner may say "I can only say it once. Do what you think I said." If the child still does not attempt the task, the examiner moves on to the next item. After the child performs a command, tokens should be moved back to their original positions. Whereas the adult administration of the Token Test makes allowances for initial inattention by allowing repetition of items in Part I, the children's administration does not.

Each correct response earns one point, so that the highest possible score is 61. When scoring it is important that the clinician note, among other things, whether the child makes the distinction between instructions such as "touch" and "pick-up" as directed in the latter portions of the test.

TABLE 11-4 Token Test Commands

Part I
(Large squares and circles only are on the table.)
1. Touch the red circle.
2. Touch the green square.
3. Touch the red square.
4. Touch the yellow circle.
5. Touch the blue circle.
6. Touch the green circle.
7. Touch the yellow square.
8. Touch the white circle.
9. Touch the blue square.
10. Touch the white square.

Part II
(Large and small squares and circles are on the table.)
1. Touch the small yellow circle.
2. Touch the large green circle.
3. Touch the large yellow circle.
4. Touch the large blue square.
5. Touch the small green circle.
6. Touch the large red circle.
7. Touch the large white square.
8. Touch the small blue circle.
9. Touch the small green square.
10. Touch the large blue circle.

TABLE 11-4 Continued

Part III
(Large squares and circles only are on the table.)
1. Touch the yellow circle and the red square.
2. Touch the green square and the blue circle.
3. Touch the blue square and the yellow square.
4. Touch the white square and the red square.
5. Touch the white circle and the blue circle.
6. Touch the blue square and the white square.
7. Touch the blue square and the white circle.
8. Touch the green square and the blue circle.
9. Touch the red square and the yellow circle.
10. Touch the red square and the white circle.

Part IV
(Large and small squares and circles are on the table.)
1. Touch the small yellow circle and the large green square.
2. Touch the small blue square and the small green circle.
3. Touch the large white square and the large red square.
4. Touch the large blue square and the large red square.
5. Touch the small blue square and the small yellow circle.
6. Touch the small blue circle and the small red circle.
7. Touch the large blue square and the large green square.
8. Touch the large blue circle and the large green circle.
9. Touch the small red square and the small yellow circle.
10. Touch the small white square and the large red square.

Part V
(Large squares and circles only are on the table.)
1. Put the red circle on the green square.
2. Put the white square behind the yellow circle.
3. Touch the blue circle with the red square.
4. Touch—with the blue circle—the red square.
5. Touch the blue circle and the red square.
6. Pick up the blue circle or the red square.
7. Put the green square away from the yellow square.
8. Put the white circle in front of the blue square.
9. If there is a black circle, pick up the red square.
10. Pick up the squares, except the yellow one.
11. When I touch the green circle, you take the white square.
12. Put the green square beside the red circle.
13. Touch the squares slowly and the circles quickly.
14. Put the red circle between the yellow square and the green square.
15. Except for the green one, touch the circles.
16. Pick up the red circle—No!—the white square.
17. Instead of the white square, take the yellow circle.
18. Together with the yellow circle, take the blue circle.
19. After picking up the green square, touch the white circle.
20. Put the blue circle underneath the white square.
21. Before touching the yellow circle, pick up the red square.

From DiSimoni, D. (1978). *The Token Test for Children: Manual.* New York: DLM-Teaching Resources. Reprinted with permission.

Detailed scoring criteria are provided in the test manual as are normative data for children age 3 through 12.5 years (DiSimoni, 1978), The adult form of the test can be used with individuals older than 12.5 years.

On each of the five sections of the test, the child must respond to the examiner's verbal commands by a motor response. Parts I–IV are composed of directions of increasing length requiring retention of two to six bits of information. The task demands are altered on Part V so that the child is required to decode syntactically and semantically complex commands. The task involves auditory processing and decoding, auditory memory, and motor planning. The relative contributions of the skills necessary for adequate performance on each section may vary somewhat. Part IV appears to more heavily assess sequential memory whereas Part V more heavily taps syntactic and semantic processing. Certain subtypes of language-disordered children may perform adequately on Part V, in which the redundancy provided by the syntax is useful, and increasingly less proficiently on Parts I–IV, in which auditory sequential memory is more critical. The opposite pattern, that is, proficiency on Part IV and poor performance on Part V, is common among children with auditory semantic comprehension problems.

Peabody Picture Vocabulary Test-Revised

The Peabody Picture Vocabulary Test-Revised (PPVT-R) (Dunn & Dunn, 1981) is another test instrument that can be easily administered as a part of a screening battery. The test has been designed to offer an index of the child's receptive vocabulary skills. The experienced clinician also can make a number of inferences about the rest of the child's receptive language functioning based on the child's performance on the test. The test is particularly good to use with children who are nonverbal due to an acquired injury, or those who are simply reluctant to speak for any reason.

As an added "bonus," one of the derived scores from the PPVT-R is a standard score based on a scale with a mean of 100 and standard deviation of 15 points, the same basic standard score scale as that used for the Wechsler Intelligence Scales. Research has shown that the PPVT-R (and its precursor, the PPVT) correlates fairly highly with Wechsler scale Verbal IQ measures and somewhat less well with the Full Scale IQ derived from the Wechsler scales (Dunn & Dunn, 1981). Thus, an estimate of the child's overall intellectual capacity can be derived. In those situations where available time precludes administering a complete Wechsler Intelligence Scale, the PPVT-R can be substituted to attain a rough but reasonably accurate estimate.

The PPVT-R is administered by asking the child to either point to, or give the number of, the one picture of four alternatives presented to the child that best represents the word said by the examiner. After establishing the required basal level of performance (eight consecutive correct responses), the test continues until the child meets the criterion for discontinuing the test (six incorrect responses in eight consecutive items). Approximate starting points are provided based on the age of the child which help to keep total administration time to a minimum.

Speech Sounds Perception Test

The Speech Sounds Perception Test is another screening test that can be used when attempting to assess language functions in children. Because of the need for some reading skills to take the test, it can be used only with individuals *age 9 and older.* Essentially, it is a test of auditory perception that assesses the child's ability to discriminate between similar sounding consonants. The tests consists of 60 multiple-choice items. The child listens to a nonsense word on tape and must choose among three alternative spellings of the word (the adult version has four alternatives). All words have the same internal vowel sound ("ee") and differ only in the beginning and ending consonant sound. Poor performance on this test tends to reflect limited concentration, poor discriminative hearing, or an inability to match visual and auditory information. Comparatively recent research suggests that a shortened version of the Speech Sounds Perception Test (30 items versus 60 items in the full test) may yield the same information in roughly one-half the administration time (Moehle, Berg, Lancaster, & Huck, 1985).

Identification of Objects by Use

Another quick test of intact language can be achieved by having the child identify common objects by their use as a means to identify the presence of an ideational dyspraxia. This type of task is a commonly found feature in comprehensive language assessment batteries (e.g., Eisensen, 1954; Porch, 1971). One study of the incidence of ideational dyspraxia in adults found that about 34% of aphasic patients were unable to identify the use of objects (DeRenzi, Pieczuro, & Vignolo, 1968). These findings suggest that *this technique can be readily used in a rapid screening for language difficulties in children as long as it is remembered that although failure on such a task increases the likelihood of an associated language disorder, success does not rule out the presence of verbal difficulties. In addition, poor performance on such a task by a child does not have the potential for localization of a lesion in children that exists in adults.*

SCREENING FOR VERBAL FLUENCY

A large number of children with acquired aphasia will experience changes in speed and fluency of verbal production. In children, greatly reduced verbal production almost always accompanies most forms of language disorder, but *it does not necessarily indicate the presence of aphasia* since a number of other childhood problems can lead to decreased verbal production. Impaired verbal fluency is also associated with damage to the frontal regions of the brain, particularly the left frontal region anterior to Broca's area (Benton, 1968; Milner, 1967).

Verbal fluency problems may be manifested in speech, reading, or writing. In children, it will affect all three activities more often than not. A number of techniques exist for quickly checking verbal fluency during the course of a screening for possible brain dysfunction. All of the tests noted in this section can be used to evaluate both younger and older children as well as adults.

Word Naming

One of the earliest verbal fluency tests, Word Naming, requires the child to say as many words as possible in one minute, but not in sentences or number series. In Terman and Merrill's 1960 standardization of the Stanford–Binet Intelligence Test, 59% of the 10-year-olds tested gave a minimum of 28 words, which was considered normal for that age. This standard can act as a rough guide in the evaluation of the child's performance. If the clinician has the recently revised version of the Stanford–Binet Intelligence Test, normative data are available for a large portion of the age range the clinician is likely to be asked to evaluate.

Boston Naming Test

The Boston Naming Test (Kaplan, Goodglass, & Weintraub, 1978) consists of 85 large pen-and-ink drawings of items ranging in familiarity from such common ones as tree and pencil at the beginning of the test to sphinx and trellis at the end (Lezak, 1983). When the child is unable to name a drawing, the examiner gives a stimulus clue. For example, if the child is unable to name a drawing, a phonetic clue is provided—for pelican, "it's a bird," "pe." The examiner keeps track of how often clues are needed and which ones are successful. Age-graded norms for adults based on a normal population are avilable (Borod, Goodglass, & Kaplan, 1980) are available that can be extended downward for children. Although the test was originally designed for the evaluation of naming deficits, Kaplan notes that it is useful for evaluation of patients with right hemisphere damage, as some of the drawings may elicit responses reflective of perceptual fragmentation.

Story Telling as a Screening for Expressive Disorders

Pictures offer a good standard stimulus for eliciting verbal production in child. The Birthday Party picture from the Stanford–Binet Intelligence scales (Terman & Merrill, 1973) can be used for this purpose. The picture is simply presented to the child and he is asked to describe what is happening in the scene depicted. Reponses to the picture provide information about how effectively the child perceives and integrates the elements of the picture (Lezak, 1982) and about such aspects of verbal ability as choice of words, vocabulary level, knowledge of syntax and grammar, and the richness and complexity of the child's statements. Other good pictures that can be used for this type of task include the Cookie Theft Picture from the Boston Diagnostic Aphasia Examination (Goodglass & Kaplan, 1979) and the Smashed Window picture developed by Wells and Ruesch (1969). The Cookie Theft picture is good for sampling propositional speech as the simple line drawing depicts familiar characters (a mother, a boy) engaged in familiar activities (washing dishes) in a common setting (a kitchen). The Smashed Window picture requires the child to appreciate social cues and integrate a number of discrete stimuli to make sense out of the scene in the picture.

Controlled Word Association Test

The production of spoken words beginning with a designated letter has been studied a great deal by a number of researchers (e.g., Benton, 1973). The associative value of each letter of the alphabet, with the exceptions of X and Z, was determined in a normative study using control subjects who were not brain injured (Borowski, Benton, & Spreen, 1967). Control subjects of low ability were found to perform less well than brighter brain-damaged patients. This result highlights the need to account for the child's premorbid verbal skills when evaluating verbal fluency.

The Controlled Word Association Test consists of three-word naming trials using the letters F, A, and S, respectively. The examiner asks the child to say as many words as he can think of that begin with the given letter of the alphabet, excluding proper nouns, numbers, and the same word with a different suffix. The score is the sum of all correct words pronounced in the three one-minute trials, adjusted for age, sex, and education. The adjusted scores can then be converted to percentiles.

ACADEMIC SKILLS

Few common neuropsychological tests or batteries of tests contain tests of learned verbal skills such as reading, writing, spelling, and arithmetic. However, impairment in these important childhood activities can have a profound impact on the child's academic success. A child's performance can also provide clues to the nature of the underlying organic dysfunction. Thus, any good screening for brain impairment should contain at least a quick assessment of a child's academic achievement. It becomes quite important that the child's premorbid academic performance level be determined to ascertain the approximate degree of dysfunction. Unlike the assessment of adults, where certain minimum assumptions of academic skills competence can be assumed by knowledge of the last grade attended in conjunction with the individual's premorbid work history, the pre-existing database of acquired information in a child of a given age is far less. Reasonable estimates of a child's premorbid academic competence can be determined by examining the child's academic records and by talking with his teacher(s).

Reading

Boder's (1973) Diagnostic Screening Procedure

This simple test was originally designed for diagnosing developmental dyslexia and can be useful in analyzing reading disorders associated with acquired brain injuries in children. All materials needed for administering it are given in the original article by Boder (1973). The first section of the test contains eight 20-word lists graded in order of difficulty from pre-primer (e.g., "go") to sixth grade (e.g., "earthquake") reading levels. The child's responses are scored according to speed. Responses made within one second of exposure receive credit for what is referred to as "flash" recognition and then the child is shown the next word. Words correctly read within 10 seconds earn "untimed" credit. "Flash" recognition words are considered to be a part of the child's sight vocabulary. The highest grade level at which 50 or more words are read by sight is the child's reading level. To determine the extent to which the child reads by sight or phonetically, the clinician only needs to compare the number of "flash" and "untimed" words that the child reads correctly.

The second section of the Diagnostic Screening Procedure is a spelling test that comes in two parts, "known" words from the sight vocabulary and "unknown" words that are not a part of the sight vocabulary. The clinician first dictates 10 words from the three highest grades of the sight vocabulary for spelling by the child. Next, 10 "unknown" words at the child's grade level or higher are dictated. Analyses of the child's performance focuses on the relative number of phonetic and nonphonetic "known" words correctly spelled and on the effectiveness of phonetic spelling of "unknown" words by the child.

Boder has defined three classifications of childhood dyslexia, all of which are characterized by reversals and letter-order errors:

1. *Dysphonetic Dyslexics.* These children have the capacity for immediate recognition and fluent reading of a limited number of words; their sight vocabulary which they read "globally as instantaneous gestalts." Such children are unable to read or spell phonetically but are able to spell known words that they can visualize. The reading and spelling of this group of children are characterized by conceptually related word substitutes.

2. *Dyseidetic Dyslexics.* This group of children are described by Boder (1973) as "letter blind" in that they have difficulty in learning to distinguish letters due to a deficit in forming visual gestalts. Once these children have learned to associate sounds with letter forms, they read by phonetic analysis and develop little, or no, sight vocabulary. Their greatest difficulty, thus, comes in attempting to read nonphonetic words. Spelling errors are phonetic but not bizarre. The children in this grouping generally misspell phonetic words that they know by sight but spell unknown phonetic words correctly.

3. *Mixed Dysphonetic–Dyseidetic Dyslexics (Alexia).* This group of children have the greatest difficulty as would be expected. These children are unable to effectively use either sight or sound readily and have difficulty with all apsects of reading and spelling.

General Academic Screening Batteries

Peabody Individual Achievement Test

The Peabody Individual Achievement Test (PIAT; Dunn & Markwardt, 1970) is a norm referenced, individually administered academic achievement screening instrument that samples from five areas of basic academic skills—mathematics, reading recognition, reading comprehension, spelling, and general information. It can be used with children from kindergarten through high-school age. Average administration time is about 30 minutes. All items in each of the academic skills subtests are presented in increasing order of difficulty. As with the PPVT mentioned earlier, a basal level of performance is established with assessment continuing until the child reaches the criteria for discontinuing each of the subtests.

The wide coverage of achievement levels makes this test useful for assessing residual competency in brain-injured children. The PIAT primarily assesses verbal conceptual functions; however, the stimulus material, being mostly visual—both verbal and visual in content—allows for an indirect assessment of a variety of a number of visual-perceptual functions as well (Lezak, 1983). Since the test requires no complex motor responding, it is a good choice for physically handicapped children.

The Mathematics subtest is a multiple-choice test on which only a pointing response is necessary. It begins with simple symbol and number recognition and ends with algebra and geometry problems. The Reading Recognition subtest is structured so that on the first nine items, the child can respond by pointing, with verbal responses required thereafter. Items 10 to 17 assess single-letter recognition and the remaining items call for correct pronunciation of increasingly difficult words ranging from "run" and "play" to "apophthegm." The third subtest, Reading Comprehension, requires the child to select which of four drawings is described in a printed sentence that is read silently by the child. The Spelling subtest also is multiple choice in format and covers the full range of difficulty levels. Items 1 through 14 assess letter and word recognition while the remainder of the items are structured so that the child must select the correct spelling of the target word from four alternative spellings. The last subtest, General Information, is a question-and-answer subtest of knowledge of common information.

Each subtest consists of 84 items except for Reading Comprehension, which has 66. Each subtest has its own normative data and scores can be converted to a wide range of standard scores such as percentiles for each age and grade level, grade equivalents, and age equivalents. Each subtest can be administered as part of the entire battery or individually depending on the clinician's need.

Wide Range Achievement Test-Revised

The Wide Range Achievement Test-Revised (WRAT-R) (Jastak & Wilkinson, 1984) provides an estimate of a child's individual academic achievement. The test has had numerous revisions since its introduction in 1936. The most recent revision has resulted in some changes in items and has used more sophisticated scaling techniques than the earlier versions. The WRAT-R assesses reading recognition, spelling, and arithmetic skills. There are two distinct tests in the WRAT-R. Level I was designed for ages 5 years, 0 months through 11 years, 11 months whereas Level II assesses skills in individuals ages 12 years and older.

The Level I spelling test is in three parts—copying a short set of nonsense figures, writing one's name, and spelling to dictation. The Level II spelling to dictation differs only in the difficulty of the words to be spelled by the child. Both Arithmetic Levels have two parts, an orally administered section for

Verbal Screening Instruments

those at the lowest level of the test and a written arithmetic test for which the child is allowed 10 minutes to complete as many items as he is able. Reading for Level I starts with letter reading and recognition and continues with a 75-word reading and pronunciation list. Level II reading involves only the word list. Administration time averages about 20–25 minutes.

Specific test items are scored objectively as either correct or incorrect with the resulting raw scores converted into grade equivalents, standard scores, and percentiles. The standard scores are, perhaps, more accurate (Gabel et al., 1986) as the grade ratings tend to be a bit inflated and/or otherwise inaccurate for many groups. Since the standard scores are structured along the same scoring scale as the Wechsler scales and other common tests (mean = 100; standard deviation = 15), direct comparisons of a child's performance on the WRAT-R to that on other tests is possible.

The WRAT-R's greatest utility arises in situations where an academic screening is necessary. When the WRAT-R standard scores differ significantly from standard IQ test scores or when there is significant variability among the three WRAT-R standard scores, possible cognitive dysfunction may be indicated and a referral for more complete evaluation may be required.

The Reading and Spelling subtests of the WRAT-R are highly verbal in nature. The Arithmetic subtest can be valuable in screening because of the variety of mathematical problems it poses (Lezak, 1983). These include application of the four basic arithmetic operations to two- and three-digit numbers, decimals, percentages, fractions, and so on. Thus, when a child's mathematical performance is deficient, the clinician can often determine by examining the child's worksheet whether his difficulties are due to a dyscalculia of the spatial type, difficulty in recognizing symbols or numbers, or a more basic loss or knowledge of number concepts or basic operations.

Many children are unable to complete more than a few arithmetic problems within the 10-minute time limit; however, the examiner has the option of simply noting how much of the test the child completes in 10 minutes and allowing the child to continue to work until he has completed all that he can. This procedure, if time allows, will enable the clinician to get a more complete picture any specific difficulties the child may have with arithmetic.

12
Screening Children for Memory Functions

Memory cannot be considered a unitary construct. Therefore, a screening of memory functioning in children should cover the span of immediate memory, the addition of new information to recent memory, the extent of recent memory, and the capacity of the individual for new learning (Lezak, 1983). Ideally, these different memory functions would be systematically reviewed through the major input and output modalities with both recall and retrieval techniques. However, in situations where memory deficiencies do not appear to be the primary problem for the child, thoroughness can be sacrificed for a number of practical considerations such as available time and maintaining the child's cooperation, and fatigue.

With most children, the Wechsler Intelligence Scale for Children-Revised (WISC-R; Wechsler, 1974) generally is a good starting point. It directly enables the clinician to assess the span of immediate memory as well as the extent of remote memory (via the Information subtest) stored in verbal form. The long Arithmetic and Comprehension subtest questions also can offer the clinician incidental information on the duration and stability of the immediate verbal memory trace. The Child Mental Status Examination (described in Chapter 7) can act to augment information gathered from the child with a delayed verbal memory task requiring the child to recall spoken items after a period of intervening material, as well as with questions to assess the retention of ongoing experience at a minimal necessary level. The addition of an immediate memory and retention measure, using simple designs, and a test of learning ability will offer more complete review of the major dimensions and modalities of memory functioning.

When performance of these types of tasks is not significantly depressed relative to the child's best performance on other tasks, and particularly when performance on tests of remote memory is not significantly better than the handling of learning tasks, the clinician can make the assumption that learning and memory are reasonably intact. Pronounced difficulties noted during a general review of memory functions may point to the need for a more in-depth memory assessment involving the systematic comparison of between functions; modalities; and the length, type, and complexity of content.

A relatively poor performance only on tests of immediate memory and learning may indicate that the child is depressed, possibly physically ill, has been exposed to some form of environmental toxin, or may have ingested some low-level toxic substance such as lead paint chips, for example. This result may point to the need for a differential diagnosis. Impaired immediate memory and learning are also common symptoms of a variety of neurological conditions that may lead to a general decline in cognitive abilities. As has been noted elsewhere in this text, brain injury in children, particularly those who are young, more often leads to a generalized decline in cognitive capabilities than to isolated deficits.

VERBAL MEMORY AND LEARNING PROBLEMS

A number of techniques can be used to screen children for the presence of verbal memory and learning problems. The almost unlimited possibilities for combining different kinds of verbal stimuli with input and output modalities and presentation formats have led to an explosion of verbal memory tests. Unfortunately, comparatively few have data concerning the performance of children, although with the rapid growth of the field of pediatric/child clinical neuropsychology, more such tests are becoming available all the time. Many of the tests for verbal memory functioning have been developed in response to specific clinical problems or research questions. Only a few have received enough use or sufficiently careful standardization to have reliable normative data. Moreover, because of the lack of systematic comparisons between different verbal memory tests, their relative utility and potential interchangeability are actually unknown. For this reason, the discussion will be limited to those few tests that have been demonstrated to be useful to the clinician.

In working with a child, the choice of memory screening tests will depend on clinical judgment in many instances rather than on scientific demonstration that any given test is most suitable for answering a specific question. Even with the number of tests available, the examiner may periodically find that none will suit the needs of a specific child, and he may be required to devise his own individual memory test for screening purposes.

Digit Span

The Digit Span subtest of the WISC-R (Wechsler, 1974) is one of the more widely used tests of verbal immediate memory. The test has two general sections, both consisting of seven pairs of random sequences of numbers. In the Digits Forward segment, the examiner reads aloud number sequences that are from three to nine digits long, and the child must repeat each sequence exactly as it is heard. The Digits Backward section of the subtest operates in much the same fashion with sequences ranging in length from two to eight digits. The major difference between the two sections is that on the Digits Backward segment the child must repeat the digits read by the examiner in reverse order. Each section of Digit Span is discontinued when the child fails to repeat both number sequences of a pair of equal length.

Three scores are produced by the test: Digits Foward, Digits Backward, and total Digit Span. The Forward and Backward scores are the number of digits in the longest correctly repeated sequence for each section. The total Digit Span score is the sum of the scores of the two sections. Most children in the age range covered by the test (ages 6–16) are able to recall at least four digits foward and three backward, but fewer than 1% are able to retain and recall the maximum nine forward and eight backward. The number of digits, both forward and backward, a child is able to retain and recall will vary with the age of the child, but the average adult will be able to recall six digits forward and five backward. Most average children are able to attain this performance by the age of 12–14 years.

In addition to immediate-auditory verbal memory, Digit Span involves auditory attention. The Digits Backward segment of the test measures not only immediate memory, but also the capacity of the child to juggle information mentally. The ability to reverse sequences effectively requires both memory and the reversing operation to operate simultaneously, a kind of mental "double tracking" (Lezak, 1983). That Digits Forward and Digits Backward do not involve identical operations is apparent in the score discrepancy of three or more points between the Forward and Backward segments that tends to occur in brain-injured individuals with concentration problems. Such performance is common in brain-damaged children but not in children who do not demonstrate difficulties with concentration (Costa, 1975).

Because of its memory and attention components, Digit Span remains one of the WISC-R subtests most sensitive to the effects of any kind of brain injury. *As a general rule, a difference of three or more points between Digits Forward and Digits Backward reflects a concentration deficit that may be of organic origin, and any Digits Forward score of four or less is suggestive of impaired immediate memory.* Digit span scores tend to be the lowest immediately following brain injury and generally increase over time, although the scores may remain low in relation to other subscale scores even several years post injury (Reitan & Davison, 1974)

The K-ABC (Kaufman & Kaufman, 1983), the Stanford–Binet Intelligence Test (Thorndike, Hagen, & Sattler, 1986, and the Illinois Test of Psycholinguistic Abilities (Kirk, McCarthy, & Kirk, 1968) also have variations of the Digit Span test that can be used to assess immediate auditory memory function of younger children (under 6 years of age.)

Rey Auditory-Verbal Learning Test

This is an easily administered test that measures immediate memory span, provides a learning curve, elicits tendencies toward retroactive and proactive interference, assesses confusion or confabulation on memory tasks, and measures retention following an intervening activity (Rey, 1964).

The test begins as a test of immediate word memory span. For the first trial (of six), the examiner reads a list of 15 words at the rate of one per second (see Table 12-1). Prior to beginning the list, the child is told that he will be read a word list and then asked to repeat as many as he can remember, in any order when the examiner stops. The examiner writes down the words recalled by the child in the order recalled. In this way, the child's pattern of recall can be tracked, noting whether he proceeds in a systematic manner, whether he associates two or three words, or whether the child's recall is a hit-or-miss proposition. If the child asks whether a word has already been said, he should be told; however, this information should not be volunteered, since it may distract the child and interefere with performance.

TABLE 12-1 Rey Auditory-Verbal Learning Test Words

List A	List B	List C
Drum	Desk	Book
Curtain	Teacher	Flower
Bell	Bird	Train
Coffee	Shoe	Rug
School	Stove	Meadow
Parent	Mountain	Harp
Moon	Glasses	Salt
Garden	Towel	Finger
Hat	Cloud	Apple
Farmer	Boat	Chimney
Nose	Lamb	Button
Turkey	Gun	Key
Color	Pencil	Dog
House	Church	Glass
River	Fish	Rattle

When the child indicates that no additional words can be recalled, the examiner gives a second set of instructions and then rereads the list. The second instruction set informs the child that the same list will be read again and that, when it is completed, the child is to say back as many words as can be remembered. The child is also asked to repeat the words said the first time and told that the order is not important. The second set of instructions must emphasize the inclusion of the previously said words so that the child does not think that the test is one of elimination.

The list is reread for trials 3, 4, and 5, using the second set of instructions each time. Praise may be given as words are recalled, and the child may be told the number of words recalled, particularly if he is able to use this information for reassurance or as a challenge. On the completion of the last trial, the second word list is read, with instructions similar to those used for the first word list. Following the reading of the second list, the child is asked to recall as many words from the first list as he can (trial VI). Should either the first or second presentations of the list be spoiled by interruptions, improper administration, confusion, or premature response on the child's part, a third word list is available.

The score for each trial is the number of words correctly recalled. A total score, the sum of trials one through five, can also be calculated. Words that are repeated can be noted, as can words that were not on the list (errors or confabulations). Normative data are available for this test that can be used with children aged 6 years and older. Talley (1987) has reported reference data for learning disabled children ranging in age from 7 to 16 years for short-term and long-term memory (see Table 12-2).

TABLE 12-2 Means and SDs for the Rey Auditory Verbal Learning Test

Age	N	Short-Term	Long-Term
7	18	12.3 (2.5)	34.7 (6.1)
8	18	13.2 (4.1)	36.4 (11.3)
9	34	14.1 (3.3)	41.4 (9.4)
10	24	15.2 (3.3)	45.1 (10.2)
11	20	16.2 (3.5)	46.7 (10.2)
12	13	16.2 (4.7)	43.8 (13.3)
13	9	15.3 (3.7)	49.1 (8.9)
14–16	17	16.8 (4.9)	45.6 (12.9)
Total	153	14.8 (3.9)	42.4 (11.0)

These data do not represent normative data and should be used by the examiner only as a rough guideline as to the performance which can be expected by this group. Short-term groupings is the sum of trials one and two and the interference trial. Long-term grouping is the sum of trials three to five, immediate recall and delayed recall. SD values are in parentheses.

Talley, J. L. (1986). Memory in learning disabled children: Digit span and the Rey Auditory Verbal Learning Test. *Archives of Clinical Neuropsychology, 1,* 315–322. Reproduced by permission.

Paired Associates Tasks

Studies with paired associates learning and related tasks have provided some insight into the difficulties that children have with some memory tasks. In this type of task that assesses verbal retention, the child is typically asked to learn 10 word pairs, about half of which form "easy," that is, meaningful, associations (e.g., read–book) and the remainder form "hard" word pairs that are not readily associated (e.g., glass–tree). The list is read several times (the average is three), with a memory trial following each reading. The total score is the number of word pairs learned, usually with different weights assigned to the "easy" and "hard" word pairs.

A variety of this type of task is readily available to the clinician, the most common of which can be found in the Wechsler Memory Scale-Revised (Wechsler & Stone, 1987). [It should be noted that, as of this writing, the availability of this test is limited due to production delays; however, in the near future, the WMS-R should be widely available (Psychological Corporation, personal communication, December 9, 1987). Until the test is widely available, the paired associate learning test in the original Wechsler Memory Scale (Wechsler & Stone, 1945) can be used.] Another version of this type of test can be found in the Randt Memory Test (Randt & Brown, 1983).

Both the Randt and the WMS-R are good, comprehensive test batteries that assess a variety of aspects of memory in a realtively brief period of time. Unfortunately, both test batteries are designed for individuals aged 16 years and older with no data available concerning the performance of younger individuals. For this reason, neither of the test batteries will be discussed at length here. The experienced clinician, however, may wish to make use of either of these batteries for assessing memory in children qualitatively until such time as normative data become available.

WPPSI Sentences Test

The Sentences subtest of the Wechsler Preschool and Primary Scale of Intelligence (WPPSI; Wechsler, 1967) is a measure of immediate recall and attention. The child is required to listen to sentences read orally by the clinician and then to repeat each sentence verbatim. The test consists of 13 sentences of increasing length ranging from 2 to 18 words. The test is stopped after three consecutive incorrectly repeated sentences. Errors include omissions, transpositions, additions, and word substitutions. The subtest, as is the case with the rest of the WPPSI, has been designed for administration to children from ages 4 years to 6 years, 6 months.

Since success on this test depends on verbal facility (Wechsler, 1967), poor performance may not necessarily indicate impaired memory functioning. In younger children, that is, under the age of 5 years, Lutey (1967) noted that performance may be a function of verbal comprehension and knowledge whereas for those children over the age of 5, the test probably does assess immediate verbal recall.

McCarthy Scales Verbal Memory 2

On the Verbal Memory 2 subtest of the McCarthy Scales of Children's Abilities (McCarthy, 1972), the child is asked to retell a short story immediately after hearing it. The score is the sum of the number of salient bits of information recalled. Syntax and sequential organization recalled by the child are not formally assessed and, therefore, are not reflected in this score; however, review of the child's responses, which should be noted verbatim, may offer important information about the child's expressive language skills. Th child may have difficulty in telling the story for a variety of reasons only one of which is auditory memory. Frequently, formulation and retrieval problems appear to contribute to poor performance. Although not a part of the standardized procedure, Wilson (1986) notes that difficulties that the child experiences can be probed by asking structured questions. Children with formulation problems are usually able to answer correctly, but those with memory problems are not. As is the case for all tasks presented auditorily to a child, deficits in auditory processing and/or attention can interfere with the child's performance.

McCarthy Scales Verbal Memory 1

The Verbal Memory 1 subtest of the McCarthy Scales (McCarthy, 1972) assesses retention and recall of nonredundant, nonlinguistically organized stimuli. In essence, it is similar in nature to Digit Span tests; however, the stimuli used are non-numeric. The test is a repetition task in which the child is asked to repeat two different types of stimuli: series of unrelated word sequences and sentences. Although only one summary score results from this test, differential performance on word series and sentences is common. Some children seem to have problems with sequencing and perform poorly when asked to repeat the unrelated words. However, when presented with the added contextual information provided by sentences, performance seems to be facilitated (Wilson, 1986). Functioning on this type of task may be disrupted by difficulties in auditory processing, auditory memory, sequencing, and use of expressive language. Useful information about the child's syntactic abilities may be derived from the child's errors on the sentence repetition subsection of this test.

Selective and Restricted Reminding Tests

The Selective Reminding Test is a free-recall verbal memory task designed to allow the independent and simultaneous assessment of long-term storage

Screening Children for Memory Functions

and consistent retrieval from long-term storage (Buschke, 1974a). It has been designed for used with children ages 5 years and older. Normative cutting scores are available for 5 through 8 year-olds (Buschke, 1974b) as well as 9 through 12 year-olds (Buschke, 1974a). For older children, adult versions of the test are available (Hannay & Levin, 1985).

Depending upon the version of the test used, a list of 10–12 words is read to the child at a rate of 1 every 2 seconds (see Figure 12-1). A number of alternate forms of the test are readily available (e.g., Clodfelter, Dickson, Wilkes, & Johnson, 1987). The child is then asked to recall as many words as he can in any order from the list just read to him. After each trial, the

Words	Trials											
	1	2	3	4	5	6	7	8	9	10	11	12
1. Garden												
2. Doctor												
3. Metal												
4. City												
5. Money												
6. Cattle												
7. Prison												
8. Cloth												
9. Water												
10. Cabin												
11. Tower												
12. Bottle												
Sum Recall												
Long-term Retrieval												
Short-term Recall												
Long-term Storage												
List Learning												
Random LTR												
No. of words Presented												

FIGURE 12-1 Sample Selective Reminding Form

examiner repeats all of the words the child omitted in that trial. The reminding and recall trials continue until the child has learned and recited the entire list or until 12 trials have been completed. This procedure allows the child to demonstrate learning by multiple free-recall trials without further item presentation to assess memory and learning in terms of initial storage, retention, and retrieval. On average, normal children are able to recall all 10 words of 10-word lists of animals or articles of clothing by the third or fourth trial.

A variation of this technique is called *Restricted Reminding* (Buschke & Fuld, 1974). In restricted reminding, following the first reading of the word list, the examiner again repeats those words the child did not recall and tells him to recall as many words as he can. All subsequent reminding *is limited to words not recalled on any trial.* Recall and reminding trials continue until the child has named each word on the list at least *once*. Thus, the first recall assesses immediate retention span. Spontaneous recall is demonstrated each time a word is recalled that the child has previously named. Retrieval problems becomes evident when a once-named word is recalled only sporadically thereafter. Once all the words have been named, the stability of storage can be assessed by the method of *extended recall* in which the child is given 12 more recall trials without any further reminding. The child's response can be evaluated for the number of items recalled and the consistency with which the items are recalled. Fult (1975) reported that control subjects were able to name 16/20 words on extended recall and tended to recall items consistently once they were named during the extended recall trials.

As the reader may have gathered by this point, administration of Selective and Restricted Reminding Tests can be difficult to learn. We advise against using this technique until the clinician has had a reasonable amount of practice and feels quite proficient in the administration and scoring of the tests.

VISUAL MEMORY FUNCTIONING

Most nonverbal memory tests involve visual memory. To test recall without resorting to verbalization, these tests must include a practic response, usually drawing. This, of course can serve to confound the interpretation of deficient performance, since the child's failure may arise from a practic deficit, from impaired visual or spatial memory, or from an interaction between these (and other) dysfunctions. On recognition memory tasks that do not call for a practic response, such perceptual defects as visual-spatial inattention may compound memory functioning. Therefore, the clinician must pay close attention to the quality of nonverbal memory test performance to estimate the relative contributions of memory, perceptual, and practic components to the end result of the child's performance.

To minimize the possibility of verbal mediation, most visual recall test stimuli consist of designs of nonsense figures. However, unless they are quite unfamiliar or complex, geometric designs do not fully control for verbal mediation. In addition, it is virtually impossible to design a large series of nonsense figures that do not elicit verbal associations. A number of the devices discussed below have originally been designed to be used with adults but can be used quite easily with older children.

Recognition Tests—Visual Attention Span

The Visual Attention Span subtest of the Hiskey–Nebraska Test of Learning Aptitude (Hiskey, 1966) can be used to assess the child's ability to immediately reconstruct a visual array after a brief exposure. The test was designed to be used with children ranging from 3 to 16 years of age. In this visual memory test, the child is asked to duplicate from memory a briefly viewed stimulus sequence (black and white representational pictures of common objects) from an array that increases from 6 to 18 pictures over the course of the test. The sequences to be remembered increase from one to seven items.

Visual Sequential Memory

This subtest of the ITPA (Kirk, McCarthy, & Kirk, 1968) requires the child to remember and produce visual sequences viewed briefly. The examiner exposes a picture of a given sequence of various geometric shapes to the child for 5 seconds. The stimulus card is then removed and the child is required to reproduce the sequence selecting the appropriate plastic chips from several on which the shapes are printed. Two trials are allowed per test item. The test continues until two consecutive items have been failed. This subtest was designed to assess a child's nonrepresentational memory in an attempt to reduce the influence of verbal mediation on visual memory processing.

The Recurring Figures Test

In the Recurring Figures Test, the stimulus materials consist of 20 cards on which are drawn geometric or irregular nonsense figures (Kimura, 1963). After looking at each of the cards in succession, the child is shown a deck of 140 cards, one at a time for 3 seconds each. The deck contains 7 sets of the 8 of the original 20 designs interspersed throughout the remaining 84 unique cards not previously seen by the child. The child must indicate whether a given card had already been seen. A perfect score for the test is 56. False-positive responses by the child are subtracted from the total correct response to correct for guessing. In Kimura's original study, the control subjects obtained a mean score of 38.9 when the correction for guessing was figured in.

DeRenzi (1968) developed a much shorter variant of this test. The stimulus set consists of 8 meaningless figures interspersed with 12 other nonsense figures in three 20-card sets. Identical instructions are used, as is the same scoring system including the correction for guessing. The maximum possible score is 24. The average correct score for this version of the test is 18.

Memory Subtests from the Stanford–Binet Scales

The Stanford–Binet Intelligence scales contain two simple visual recall tasks that are suitable for screening purposes, particularly with very young children—the nonverbal Delayed Response Test at age level II and the Naming Object from Memory Test at age level IV. The Delayed Response Test uses a small cat figurine and three small boxes. On each of three trials, the examiner hides the cat under a different box, screens the boxes for a count of 10, and then asks the child to point to the box hiding the cat. The naming from Memory Test uses a box and nine different small objects. On each of three trials, three of the objects are set out and named by the child, who then keeps his eyes closed while the examiner covers one of the three objects with the box. The child must then recall which object is hidden. For both tests, the child must respond correctly on at least two of the three trials to "pass" the test.

Memory for Designs

This test is similar to other types of drawing tests (such as the Bender Visual-Motor Gestalt Test), except that the designs must be drawn from memory (Graham & Kendall, 1960). This tests consists of 15 geometric designs that vary in complexity. The designs are shown to the child one at a time for 5 seconds. Immediately after each exposure, the child is asked to draw what he remembers of the design. The reproductions are scored for errors, based on a point system that awards one point for two or more errors when the essential design is preserved, two points when the configuration of the design has been lost or a major element is missing or greatly distorted, and three points for rotations and reversals. Perhaps because the original intent of the test was to screen for "organicity" and not for memory per se, no points are given for designs that have been completely forgotten. Thus, the error score of a child with extremely defective immediate recall who forgets some or all of the designs may not be significantly elevated. Conversely, the three-point penalties given to rotations and reversals elevate some childrens's scores disproportionately (Grundvig, Needham, & Ajax, 1970). For older children and young adults, the raw scores may be interpreted directly, whereas for younger individuals a correction based on age and general ability (based on the Wechsler or Stanford–Binet Vocabulary score) is recommended by the test author. In any age group, qualitative aspects of performance related to memory should be noted as well as the quantitative score which also reflects constructional ability.

The Knox Cube Test

The Knox Cube Test (Stone & Wright, 1980) was originally created to help detect cognitive impairment in immigrants who did not speak English. Its lack of reliance on verbal instructions or responses makes it attractive as an instrument to evaluate individuals such as young children who do not have advanced verbal skills. It consists of four small wooden blocks arranged linearly on a strip of plywood and a fifth loose cube. The examiner uses the loose cube to tap a sequence on the other four. The child is then asked to repeat the sequence. In the "junior" version of the test, the items range from two-cube sequences to six-cube sequences. The "senior" form overlaps with the junior form so that superior performance can be assessed further by adding the senior version items. Administrationm continues until five consecutive sequences are missed by the child.

The Knox Cube Test is primarily a measure of visual sequential memory; however, the scoring procedures allow the clinician to separate visual sequential memory deficits from attentionally based deficits. The test is normed on the basis of *Item Response Theory,* allowing scaling in *mastery units* and conversion to age equivalency scores. The total number of correct responses is summed and converted to a mastery unit score on a profile sheet. Confidence boundaries (intervals) are then drawn around the score. Inconsistent performance is allowed inside the confidence boundaries. Incorrect responses below the lower boundary or correct responses above the upper boundary indicate a degree of inconsistency more likely to be the result of attention problems than of deficits in visual sequential memory.

The Knox Cube Test was normed on a sample of 340 individuals, 179 of whom were between 3 and 14 years of age. The test–retest reliability was reported as 0.64 in a sample of adults (Sterns, 1966). The reliability of the test for children has not been evaluated to date but may have a similar value.

As well as partialing out attention difficulties from memory deficits, the Knox Cube Test has the added benefit of being both easy to administer and portable.

Benton Visual Retention Test

The Benton Visual Retention Test (BVRT) consists of three alternate but equivalent versions that may be administered under differing conditions (Benton, 1974). The conditions include simple copying and copying from memory after various delays (no delay and 15-second delay). Each version of the tests consists of 10 cards with more than one figure in the horizontal plane; most have three figures, two large and one small, with the small figure always at one side or the other. In addition to visual memory, the test is sensitive to disruptions in visual-spatial processing. By administering one form of the test with the copying instructions and one form with the memory instructions, the clinician can separate the two types of disorders.

The BVRT was designed for individuals ranging upwards from 8 years of age. Each version of the test is scored for both the number of correct designs and the number of errors. Six types of errors are possible: omissions, distortions, perseverations, rotations, misplacements (in the relative positioning of one figure to the others), and errors in size. Therefore, it is common to have more than one error per card. But the number correct and the error score norms for Administration A (the most frequently used administration consisting of a 10-second exposure and then immediate copying from memory) take into account intelligence level and age of the child.

Interpretation of the test results is relatively straightforward. Taking the age and intellectual functioning of the child into account, the clinician uses normative tables for Administration A and determines whether either score (number correct or number of errors) falls into the impaired range. Benton (1974) considers a score of two points below the number of expected correct responses to "raise the question of impairment," whereas four or more points below the expected score is viewed as a "strong indication" of impairment. Error scores are dealt with similarly. A child whose error score exceeds the expected score, based on age and intelligence, by three or more points can be suspected of being impaired, and an error score exceeding the expected level by five or more points is considered a "strong indication" of brain dysfunction. Similar scoring criteria and methods are used for the other versions of the BVRT.

BVRT errors can be tabulated by type, enabling the clinician to determine the nature of the child's problem. Impaired immediate memory or an attention disorder will likely appear mostly as a simplification or simple substitution, or omission of the designs (Lezak, 1983). Unilateral spatial neglect (rare in children) tends to appear as a consistent omission of the figure on the same side of the design. Practic deficits most often manifest as defects in the execution or organization of the designs. Rotations and consistent design distortions generally indicate a more basic perceptual problem. In somewhat older children, perseverations should alert the clinician to look elsewhere in the child's protocol for other perseverations on different tasks. Widespread perseveration may indicate a monitoring or activity control problem, whereas perseveration limited to performance on the BVRT is usually suggestive of a specific visual or immediate memory impairment in a child who may be trying to compensate for a brain-based dysfunction. In younger children, design simplification, including a disregard of size and figure placement, often represents a normal state of affairs. Therefore, the clinician should be careful not to overdiagnose problems when using this (and other) tests.

As with other tests of visual-perceptual functioning, children with right hemisphere lesions tend to do somewhat more poorly than do children with left-sided lesions. In addition, children with more posterior damage (in the parietal-occipital region) do more poorly than do those with anterior dysfunction. However, the clinician must remain cognizant of the fact that the above statements reflect only statistical associations and are not hard-and-fast rules for diagnosis from BVRT results. Also, as noted a number of times in this book, in general, brain injuries in children often result in generalized dysfunction regardless of the actual site of injury.

Rey–Osterrieth Complex Figure Test

A "complex figure" was originally devised by Rey (1941) to investigate both perceptual organization and visual memory in brain-damaged individuals. Osterrieth (1944) standardized Rey's procedure and obtained normative data from the performance of 230 normal children ranging in age from 4 to 15 years, and 60 adults in the 16-to-20 age range. Osterrieth also gathered data from a small group of adults (43) who had sustained traumatic brain damaged as well as from a few patients with endogenous brain disease.

The test consists of Rey's figure (Figure 12-2), two blank sheets of paper, and five or six colored pencils. The child is first asked to copy the figure which has been placed so that its length runs along the child's horizontal plane. The examiner watches the child's performance closely. Each time a section of the figure is completed, a different colored pencil is handed to the child, and the order of colors is noted. Time needed to complete the figure is noted, and both the figure and drawing are removed from the child's field of vision. After 3 minutes, the child is given a second sheet of paper and is asked to draw the design from memory. The time to complete

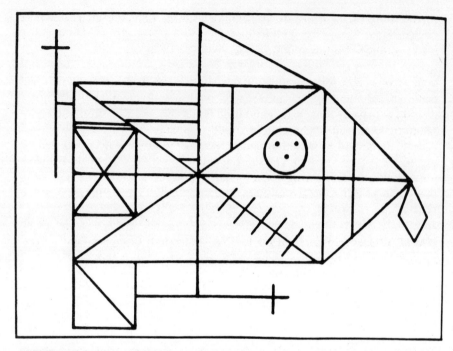

FIGURE 12-2. Rey–Osterrieth Complex Figure.

From Osterrieth, P. A. (1944). Le test de copie d'une figure complexe. *Archives de Psychologie, 30,* 206–356.

the drawing is recorded, as is whether the child follows the same procedural approach on the second drawing as on the first.

Osterrieth analyzed the drawings in terms of the method of procedure as well as specific copying errors. Seven procedural types were identified:

(1) Subject begins by drawing the large central rectangle and details are added in relation to it.
(2) Subject begins with a detail attached to the central rectangle, or with a subsection of the rectangle, completes the rectangle, and adds remaining details in relation to the rectangle.
(3) Subject begins by drawing the overall contour of the figure without explicit differentiation of the central rectangle and then adds internal details.
(4) Subject juxtaposes details one by one without an organizing structure.
(5) Subject copies discrete parts of the drawing with no semblance of organization.

Screening Children for Memory Functions

(6) Subject substitutes the drawing of a similar object, such as a boat or house.
(7) Subject produces an unrecognizable drawing.

In Osterrieth's sample, 83% of the adult control group followed procedure types 1 and 2, 15% used type 4, and one individual followed type 3. Beyond the age of 7 years, no child used types 5, 6, or 7, and from the age of 13, more than half of the children used procedure types 1 and 2.

An accuracy score, based on a unit scoring system (Table 12-3), can be obtained for each test trial. The scoring units refer to specific areas that have been numbered for scoring convenience (Figure 12-3). Since the reproduction of each unit can earn as many as 2 score points, the highest possible

TABLE 12-3 Scoring system for the Rey–Osterrieth Complex Figure Test

Units
1. Cross upper left corner, outside of rectangle
2. Large rectangle
3. Diagonal cross
4. Horizontal midline of 2
5. Vertical midline
6. Small rectangle, with 2 to the left
7. Small segment above 6
8. Four parallel lines within 2, upper left
9. Triangle above 2, upper right
10. Small vertical line within 2, below 9
11. Circle with 3 dots within 2
12. Five parallel lines with 2 crossing 3, lower right
13. Sides of triangle attached to 2 on right
14. Diamond attached to 13
15. Vertical line within triangle 13 parallel to right vertical of a
16. Horizontal line within 13, continuing 4 to right
17. Cross attached to lower center
18. Square attached to 2, lower left

Scoring
Each of the 18 units above is considered separately. Each unit is scored for accuracy and relative position within the whole of the design.

For each unit, count as follows:

Correct	Placed properly	2 points
	Placed poorly	1 point
Distorted or incomplete	Placed properly	1 point
But recognizable	Placed poorly	½ point
Absent or not recognizable		0 points
Maximum possible score		36 points

Adapted from Lezak, M. D. (1976). *Neuropsychological assessment.* New York: Oxford University Press. Copyright © 1976, Oxford University Press. Adapted by permission.

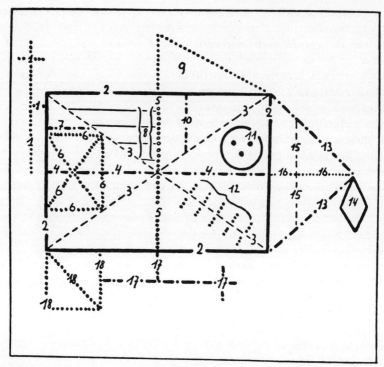

FIGURE 12-3. Scoring Units for the Rey–Osterrieth Complex Figure Test.

From Osterrieth, P. A. (1944). Le test de copie d'une figure complexe. *Archives de Psychologie, 30,* 206–356.

score is 36. The memory trial is scored in the same way. A comparison of the scores of each trial will aid the clinician in determining the presence of visuographic or visual-memory defects as well as their relative severity.

More recently, investigators have been using a somewhat modified scoring approach more suitable for younger children that allows for a more reliable and valid method for assessing those parameters most relevant for neuropsychological diagnosis and offers detailed developmental descriptive data of the child's performance (Waber & Holmes, 1985). These authors devised a scoring system for allowing quantification of the parameters of organization and style by identification of critical features (24 for organization and 18 for style) on the basis of which productions are assigned to 1 of 5 levels of organization and then categorized by style within each organizational level (Waber & Holmes, 1986). One of the basic premises of this work is that some children reproduce the design in a fragmented, part-oriented manner, whereas others use a more global or configuration-oriented manner, and that there is a "normal" developmental sequence for complex visual memory that can be tracked.

The end result of these investigations has been the development of a system that describes developmental changes in children's productions from memory of the Rey-Osterrieth figure. The authors found that total accuracy in recall was not achieved by even the oldest children in the study population, which ranged in age from 5 to 14 years. Other significant normative findings were: (1) the organizing structures (e.g., rectangle, main substructure of the figure) are remembered better at all ages; (2) material on the left side of the design is recalled better than that on the right side until the age of 8 years; (3) errors and distortions are more frequent on the memory than the copy productions at every age but are not affected by memory delay; (4) memory productions are produced more configurationally than copy productions except among the youngest children; and (5) delaying the memory production of the figure results in further loss of details and a more marked shift to the configural approach (Waber & Holmes, 1986).

Clinically, the normative findings of Waber and Holmes (1985, 1986) have a number of important implications for users of the figure. First, part-orientation in the memory production portion of the test is very rare after the age of 9, and therefore, should be viewed as significant in an older child or adult. Second, errors or distortions are relatively common in the memory condition but rare in the copy portion of the test. Errors in the copy condition and an excessive number of errors in recall, thus, are likely to indicate the presence of pathology. Finally, the findings of this research provide some insight into the development of memory for complex visual material about which little is known at present. The major finding at present is that a gestalt approach appears to predominate as individuals grow older.

These authors are continuing their research into the development of memory processes of children, and it is likely that highly significant findings will be forthcoming in the near future. (As of this writing, a test administration and scoring manual is being prepared that provides detailed instructions for using the developmental scoring system as well as normative data; however, no release date has been set.)

TACTILE MEMORY—THE TACTUAL PERFORMANCE TEST

This test uses the Sequin–Goddard Formboard, that, although originally a visuopractic task, was converted by Halstead (1947) into a tactile memory test by administering it to blindfolded subjects and adding a drawing recall segment to the test. Reitan incorporated this version of the test into his testing battery for adults. Three trials are given in Halstead's administration. Each of the first two trials is done with each hand used singly, with the preferred hand being used first. The third trial uses both hands. The score for each trial is the time to completion (getting all the blocks into the proper holes while blindfolded) in seconds. On completion of the formboard trials, and after the board and the blocks have been removed from the child's view, the blindfold is removed from the child. The child is then given a blank piece of paper and a pencil, and is instructed to draw from memory as much of the board as is remembered and to indicate the different shapes and their locations relative to one another on the board. Two scores are obtained from the drawing. The memory score is a simple count of the number of shapes reproduced with reasonable accuracy. The location score is the total number of blocks placed in proper position relative to the other shapes and the board.

Depending upon the age of the child being testing, the exact version of the board and blocks to be used will vary. For children older than 14 years, the original 10-block version of the formboard is used. If the child is between 9 and 14 years of age, a six-block version of the board is used. An eight-block formboard is also available for children in this age range since a number of investigators claim that a six-block version is too easy (e.g., Knights & Norwood, 1980). For a younger child between the ages of 5 and 8 years, the 6-block version is also used; however, the placement of the board is horizontal rather than vertical to account for the shorter reach of younger children and to allow the smaller child ample room for exploration. For each version, the child should be allowed to continue on each of the three trials until completion or a maximum of 10 minutes (per trial) has passed.

Normative data for ages five through fourteen is presented in Table 12-4 and cut-off scores for individuals older than 14 years can be seen in Table

TABLE 12-4 Tactual Performance Test Performance of Normal Subjects (Ages 5–14)

		Age								
		2–5	6	7	8	9	10	11	12	13	14
Total time	M	18.29	15.84	11.93	9.40	7.11	7.00	5.68	4.96	4.75	4.33
	SD	5.62	8.69	4.14	3.79	2.91	2.65	2.12	1.90	1.61	1.07
Memory	M	0.88	2.94	3.33	3.92	4.63	4.72	4.79	4.73	5.20	4.87
	SD	0.82	1.90	1.63	1.35	1.14	1.21	0.97	1.08	0.92	0.96
Location	M	0.21	1.26	1.77	2.48	3.29	3.42	4.27	4.03	4.05	4.42
	SD	0.44	1.52	1.76	1.63	1.71	1.69	1.36	1.30	1.28	1.23

For ages 5–8, data are for the 6 block board. For ages 9–14, data is for the 8 block formboard.

Adapted from Klonoff, H. & Low, M. (1976). Disordered brain function in young children and early adolescents: Neuropsychological and electroencephalographic correlates. In R. M. Reitan & L. A. Davison (Eds.), *Clinical neuropsychology: Current status and applications* (pp. 121–178), Washington, D.C.; V. H. Winston & Sons. Adapted with permission.

TABLE 12-5 Tactual Performance Test Cutoff Scores (Ages 15 and Older)

	Total time (min)	Memory	Location
Average performance of normal controls	10.7	6.2	5.9
Cutoff score	15.6	6.0	15.0

Data form Halstead (1947).

12-5. Although markedly slowed or defective performance on the TPT or memory trials is associated with brain damage, the nature of the organic dysfunction is not clear. Some investigators have found that individuals with right hemisphere injury perform more poorly than do those with left hemisphere injury (Reitan, 1964). However, opposite results on the recall task have also been reported (DeRenzi, 1968). Reitan (1964) considers the test to be especially sensitive to frontal lobe dysfunction.

Time difference between trials also offer important information. The difference between the time taken with the preferred hand and that taken with the nonpreferred hand may provide a clue as to the side of the lesion. There is an implicit assumption that learning will occur; thus, there should be a steady decrease in the time needed to complete the test from trial one with the preferred hand to trial three with both hands.

Part IV
SPECIAL CONSIDERATIONS IN ASSESSMENT

13
Screening Batteries for Children

SCREENING BATTERIES VERSUS SINGLE TESTS VERSUS COMPREHENSIVE TEST BATTERIES

For several years, comprehensive neuropsychological test batteries for children, such as the Reitan–Indiana, Halstead–Reitan, or Luria–Nebraska Batteries, have been shown to be effective in differentiating brain-damaged from normal children. As such, it might seem to make some degree of sense to administer a complete evaluation to every child in whom the presence of organic dysfunction is suspected. Careful evaluation of children seen in private practice, outpatient mental health clinics, or schools should identify those with brain dysfunction which will allow appropriate treatment—treatment which otherwise might not have been considered—to be instituted. However, not all clinical or school psychologists or examiners have learned the necessary skills or have had the training needed to competently administer and interpret a comprehensive neuropsychological test battery.

These skills and knowledge can readily be acquired; however, not all clinicians may be able to invest the time and money necessary to develop proficiency in the art of pediatric and child neuropsychological diagnosis and treatment planning. Much the same can be said for psychologists operating in school systems—budgetary constraints in most school systems simply do not allow for such extended additional training. Current guidelines under consideration by the American Psychological Association advise that proficiency in general (i.e., adult) neuropsychology can be attained only after a minimum of one year's exclusive and full-time postdoctoral training in neuropsychology under the supervision of a qualified neuropsychologist or through a graduate degree program with a special emphasis in neuropsychology. Expertise in the area of child or pediatric neuropsychology will require an additional, roughly equivalent period of time over and above that needed for general neuropsychology as the basic concepts and techniques of neuropsychology must be acquired before a specialty with children can be developed. At the present time, such training in general neuropsychology is not readily available throughout the country. There are comparatively few graduate training programs in psychology that offer a distinct emphasis in neuropsychology; similarly, there are few such postdoctoral training programs. The competition for the comparatively few available slots at either the pre- or postdoctoral level is keen. Specialty training in pediatric/child neuropsychology is even less common. Good pediatric/child neuropsychologists are currently a very rare breed, although the number of competent professionals practicing in this subspecialty is increasing all the time, as are available training sites.

A number of highly competent clinicians feel that they can get the requisite training by attending one or another of the workshops that have proliferated in the past several years to deal with the administration and interpretation of some of the most popular neuropsychological test batteries. However, even those who offer such workshops will admit, and frequently emphasize (the present authors included), to those in attendance that the workshop cannot make one a competent neuropsychologist. What the clinician can gain from these workshops is a knowledge of administration techniques for a given test battery as well as some very basic knowledge about interpreting the results of the test. The one-, two-, or even five-day workshop does not make the clinician expert in the plethora of complex subtleties involved in brain–behavior relationships, nor is any substantial information typically given concerning brain functions and their interrelationships that underlie manifest behaviors in either normal or brain-injured individuals. In addition, as should be evident to the reader by this point in the book, brain–behavior relationships in children are not necessarily the same as those seen when working with adults. A number of clinicians make the error of thinking that what is learned in a workshop is directly applicable to children. Such errors can have profound implications in the diagnosis of children, and in treatment and educational planning for a child with cognitive dysfunction.

A second reason that the private practice clinician or the clinician working for a school system, mental health center, or private hospital may not want to perform comprehensive neuropsychological evaluations is the sheer amount of time that is involved. In certain circumstances, a comprehensive evaluation can take up to a week, depending upon the child's physical and mental condition. More often, an evaluation will take anywhere from four to eight hours, depending on the test battery and supplemental test instruments chosen. The vast majority of practicing psychologists simply do not have that amount of time to devote to a single patient; this can be particularly true for those psychologists working for a school system. Psychologists in private practice often depend on seeing a comparatively large number of patients in any given day to earn their livelihood. For them to conduct an occasional neuropsychological evaluation that requires the devotion of a full day or more may not make economic sense. Practitioners working in mental health settings, private hospitals, or in schools may be required to see far too many children to spend the time required for a neuropsychological evaluation of one child.

Finally, the cost of equipment and materials required to conduct neuropsychological evaluations frequently can be prohibitive for only occasional use. A complete Halstead–Reitan Neuropsychological Test Battery set-up, including all equipment and associated materials, can cost close to $2,000 or more at the time of this writing. The Luria–Nebraska Neuropsychological Battery will cost roughly $300 initially. Both batteries now have computer-assisted scoring available, which can increase the cost still further, particularly if the clinician needs to purchase a computer. Thus, the initial investment can be great, and this cost does not include any additional test equipment and those materials that are frequently used by neuropsychologists to supplement the information from more comprehensive batteries. By their very nature, each of the available comprehensive evaluations, in a sense, is nothing more than a comprehensive screening battery that offers the possibility of generating hypotheses about the brain integrity of a child that may in turn require further in-depth investigation with any number of other test instruments.

In essence, to perform neuropsychological evaluations, the clinician really must be willing to devote all of her professional energies to neuropsychology. It is extremely difficult to be a good "part-time" neuropsychologist without either the general clinical practice or the neuropsychological aspect of the practice suffering. In addition, it can be quite difficult to work in both adult and pediatric/child neuropsychology. Since many of the brain–behavior relationships assessed in a typical pediatric/child neuropsychological evaluation are based on somewhat different underlying cognitive functions than those used when assessing adults, the clinician needs to be able to readily shift cognitive set back and forth between adult and child theories of cognitive functioning depending on the age of the individual being assessed.

A neuropsychological screening battery offers a practical alternative to this, since it generally does not require much in the way of special equipment. Administration and interpretation of screening batteries generally require far less time than that which is required for the more comprehensive evaluation. In addition, the cost in terms of both materials and personnel, as well as space, is typically much less. A relatively brief, portable, and easily administered and scored battery of tests is much more practical and cost effective in those situations where the primary requirement is to differentiate those children who have brain-based pathology from those who do not.

Over the years, a number of investigators have attempted to identify a single test that will differentiate patients with brain damage from non–brain-damaged individuals. In virtually all instances such attempts have failed and continue to do so. There is a very simple reason for this: One single test cannot possibly tap all aspects of brain functioning. There are individual tests that are exceptionally good in terms of identifying one or another form of organic dysfunction, such as the Halstead Category Test; however, if the child being assessed does not happen to manifest a dysfunction in the specific area of cognitive functioning being tapped by the test, but does indeed happen to have some form of cognitive impairment, that particular child may be inappropriately identified as non–brain-damaged. As a very simple example, a child with a language disturbance will likely not be identified as impaired by the Bender Visual-Motor Gestalt Test; similarly, the child with visual-spatial processing disturbance will be classified as normal if just the Speech Perception Test is used as the screening device.

A good neuropsychological screening battery is designed to minimize the time needed for administration, scoring, and interpretation while maximizing the information gathered by briefly assessing all major cognitive functional areas. These functional areas include: lateral dominance; motor functioning; auditory, tactile, and visual sensation and perception; spatial-perceptual organization; language skills; general information; and memory functioning. Furthermore, the tests included in such a screening battery should have as little redundancy as possible and should have been empirically demonstrated to be effective in differentiating brain-damaged from non–brain damaged individuals. All tests included should be brief, easily administered, objectively scored (when possible), commonly used in clinical settings, and very portable.

Unfortunately, to date there has been relatively little research conducted concerning the screening of neuropsychological functions in children as compared to that which has been done for adult screening batteries. What follows is a description of different screening batteries, a few of which are commercially available and have been reported in professional journals or discussed at length at professional meetings. The other batteries discussed are downward extensions of some of the batteries designed for adults. These have been included since all contain test instruments that tap the major areas of cognitive functions noted above, and all of the tests that comprise the batteries either have readily available versions for children or have normative data available for younger individuals.

As the experienced clinician is well aware, situations will arise where the batteries and techniques described in this chapter are inappropriate because of time constraints, lack of immediate availability of specific instruments, or other reasons. In such circumstances, the clinician may still wish to perform some form of assessment with the test instruments readily at hand. There are a tremendous number and variety of tests available for children which, when viewed from the proper perspective, can be used for determining the possible presence of particular dysfunction. Unfortunately, it is well beyond the scope of this book to discuss all of them. In this chapter, as well as in the other chapters in the book, we have attempted to describe those instruments, and combinations of instruments, which are likely to be the most useful for the general clinician. In the appendices to this book, we have compiled a listing of tests that can be used by the clinician for assessment of a variety of cognitive domains. The use of these listings, in conjunction with the information concerning cognitive functions presented throughout this text, should enable the clinician to construct her own screening battery when needed which can be reasonably effective in identifying potential brain dysfunction in a child.

WYSOCKI AND SWEET SCREENING BATTERY

The adult version of this neuropsychological screening battery was developed by Jeffrey Wysocki and Jerry Sweet (1985). The children's adaptation has been in clinical use at one of the authors' (R.B.) assessment laboratories for about $2\frac{1}{2}$ years and has been found to be useful in identifying possible cognitive impairment in children. The battery consists of seven tests and requires less than one hour for administration. In the original research investigation for the adult version of the battery, the average administration time for brain-damaged individuals was 55.6 minutes; for schizophrenic patients, 51.3 minutes; and for normal control subjects, 50.3 minutes. The time for the children's adaptation of the battery in clinical use has averaged roughly 45 minutes for brain-injured children, and about 40 minutes for both learning disabled children and child psychiatric inpatients.

The measures that make up the battery include:

1. the Finger Tapping Test (Halstead, 1947)—a measure of bilateral fine motor speed and dexterity;
2. either the Trail Making Test—Parts A and B (Armitage, 1946) for children 9–14 years of age, or the Progressive Figures Test and the Color Form Test (Reitan, 1955) for children between the ages of 5 and 9;

3. the Coding (ages 6–16) or Animal House (ages 4–6) subtests of the appropriate Wechsler Intelligence Scales—tests that assess motor persistence, sustained attention, response speed, and visual-motor coordination;
4. the Spatial Relations component—Greek Cross—of the Aphasia Screening Test (Halstead & Wepman, 1959);
5. the Pathognomonic Scale items of the Luria–Nebraska adult and children's batteries (Golden, Hammeke, & Purisch, 1985; Golden, 1987)—a series of items from the battery that have been empirically shown to be highly sensitive to the presence of cognitive dysfunction (clinically, this has been the case for a child as young as age 6 years with the children's battery despite the fact that the battery has been normed only for children between the ages of 8 and 12);
6. the Stroop Color and Word Test (Stroop, 1935);
7. the Logical Memory and Visual Reproduction sections of the Wechsler Memory Scale (Wechsler, 1945).

The Progressive Figures Tests and the Color Form Test are a part of the Reitan–Indiana Neuropsychological Test Battery for Young Children (Reitan, 1974). For the *Color Form Test*, there are geometric shapes of different colors printed on a tag board. The child is instructed to touch one figure and then another, moving in a sequence of shape–color–shape–color. The child is required to selectively attend to one aspect of the stimulus (e.g., color) and to ignore the other (e.g., shape). This test is similar to Part B of the Trail Making Test, where the child moves from numbers to letters, and back to numbers. On the *Progressive Figures Test*, there are eight large shapes (such as a circle), with smaller shapes (such as a square) inside. The child must move from the small square (inside) to a large figure with the same shape (square). The second large shape may have a smaller triangle shape inside, indicating that the next move will be a large triangular shape. This task requires visual perception, motor speed, attention, concentration, and flexibility to change sets. The rest of the tests in the battery have been discussed elsewhere in the book.

All tests are administered according to their normal instructions and scored in the standard manner described in the specific test manuals except where noted. The order in which the tests should be administered and the specific scoring criteria are presented in Table 13-1. The order was chosen by the battery developers to allow enough time to elapse between the immediate and delayed recall of the subtests from the Wechsler Memory Scale without presenting competing verbal and visual memory items found in the Pathognomonic Scale of the Luria–Nebraska Battery. The delayed recall of the Wechsler Memory scale items is obtained 20 to 30 minutes after the immediate recall portion by pausing in the administration of the

TABLE 13-1 Children's Adaptation of the Wysocki–Sweet Screening Battery: Order of Administration and Special Scoring Considerations

Test	Scoring
1. Finger tapping	The relevant measures are the mean number of taps of the index finger of each hand.
2. Wechsler Memory Scale	Immediate and one-half hour delay scores described by Russell (1975) are used for both the Logical Memory and Visual Reproduction subtests.
3. Trail Making (ages 9 and up)	The number of seconds required to complete each part.
Progressive Figures (ages 5–8)	The number of seconds required for completion of the test.
Color Form Test (ages 5–8)	The number of errors and the time (in seconds) required for completion of the test.
4. Coding (ages 6–16)	The number of correctly drawn symbols in 120 seconds.
Animal House	The number of correctly placed pegs within the maximum time limit of 5 minutes.
5. Stroop Color and Word Test	The age-corrected raw score of the number of items correctly finished in 45 seconds on each page of the Golden (1978) version.
6. Pathognomonic Scale	Summary score for the scale obtained by adding the rating scores for each of the items on the scale. (For children younger than age 8, the scoring criteria for age 8 is used.)
7. Spatial Relations (ages 6 and up)	The Greek Crosses drawn by the child are scored using the rating scale developed by Russell, Neuringer, & Goldstein (1970).

Luria–Nebraska items. The remaining Pathognomonic scale item are then administered, followed by the drawing of the Greek Crosses to complete the battery. On completion of the battery, the child's performance on each measure is compared to the traditional cutoff scores (where available) for each of the tests; if the child is impaired on six of the eight measures, she can be considered to be cognitively impaired. With adults, the "six out of eight" decision rule correctly classified 68% of the brain-damaged subjects, 84% of the schizophrenic patients as non–brain-damaged, and 100% of the normal control subjects in the original sample studied by Wysocki and Sweet (1985).

In clinical use, the children's adaptation of this battery has yielded approximately the same percentages for children over the age of 12. For younger children, to date the battery has correctly classified 122 out of 167 children with confirmed (by CT scan, MRI scan, or neurosurgical results) brain damage, and 96 out of 110 learning disabled and psychiatric children.

The children's adaptation of the Wysocki and Sweet Screening Battery appears to be a useful screening device. It meets the criteria of brevity, ease of administration, and coverage of a broad base of neuropsychological skills and cortical functions necessary for a useful screening instrument.

Of note is the fact that this battery, as good as it may be, was not able to correctly classify 45 brain-injured children. This points out a problem with neuropsychological screening batteries in general—there can be a substantial number of false negatives. Often, children will have very subtle or highly specific deficits that a screening battery will be unable to detect. The astute clinical observer may be able to improve slightly on this figure; however, there are bound to be some impaired children who will not be identified. In such instances, the best strategy for the clinician is to refer for comprehensive evaluation or neuropsychological functioning those children whose screening results are suspicious but who do not meet the criteria necessary to suggest cortical dysfunction.

FLORIDA KINDERGARTEN SCREENING BATTERY

The Florida Kindergarten Screening Battery (FKSB) was designed for the early identification (in kindergarten) of learning deficits of children (Satz & Fletcher, 1982). The manual for the battery notes that the battery has the quite restricted goal of predicting the "likelihood that an individual kindergarten child will manifest learning problems 3 years later (end of grade 2)" (Satz & Flectcher, 1982, p. 1).

The FKSB consists of four individually administered tests and requires about one hour to administer. The tests include a Recognition-Discrimination measure, an Alphabet Recitation Test, an optional supplementary measure (included with the battery), a Finger Localization Test, and two previously published tests—The Peabody Picture Vocabulary Test-Revised (PPVT-R) and the Beery Developmental Test of Visual-Motor Integration (DVMI). The battery can be administered in either the four- or five-test version with little training by an experienced technician. Complete scoring criteria and normative data are provided with the test kit. If the clinician already has the PPVT and/or the DVMI, the kit can be acquired without these two tests.

The FKSB was developed from a longitudinal study that was devised as a large-scale multivariate prediction study designed to investigate the neuropsychological factors associated with reading success and failure in elementary school children (Fletcher, Satz, & Morris, 1982; Satz, Taylor, Friel, & Fletcher, 1978). With the emphasis on neuropsychological prediction, the investigation demonstrated that it was possible to predict second-grade reading achievement levels from the tests of the FKSB given at the beginning of kindergarten.

The KFSB predicts classification according to a range of possible predicted and actual outcome categories rather than presence or absence of dysfunction. The use of these graded outcome categories (i.e., severe, mild, average, and superior) eliminates the typical overemphasis on hit rates used in screening tests (such as those reported for the children's adaptation of the Wysocki–Sweet battery discussed earlier) and provides, on a longitudinally based predictive basis, much more clinically meaningful information.

The standardization of the battery was conducted on a complete sample of 479 males who entered kindergarten in 1970 in one county in Florida. The prediction equations were derived from the collapsing of the data from the original longitudinal sample with the results of a study of 181 similar males. Gates (1984) noted that the standardization sample is fairly restricted, i.c., white, middle to upper class males) which may limit the generalizability of the results. However, reliability studies conducted on the FKSB which are reported in the manual indicate that the battery tends to have a generally high reliability. It should be noted that some authors (e.g., Gates, 1984) have criticized the battery since reliabilities for all of the tests that comprise the battery are not reported.

Overall, the FKSB is a neuropsychological screening battery with a fairly restricted goal—to predict reading or learning failure in grade two from a neuropsychological test administered to the preschool-aged child. Tupper (1986) notes that the battery performs this task reasonably well. If this is the primary reason for seeing the child, the FKSB can be considered a good choice by the clinician; however, it is not as comprehensive a screening procedure as some of the others available to, or that can be devised by, the clinician.

THE MCCARTHY SCREENING TEST

The McCarthy Screening Test (MST; McCarthy, 1978) is a preschool screening instrument for children between the ages of 4 and $6\frac{1}{2}$ years. Total administration time is about 20–25 minutes with little training required on the part of the examiner. The MST was designed to be a general screening instrument that identifies a child as developing at a slower rate than her peers. The MST thus classifies children into a "not-at-risk" or an "at-risk" for school problems group based on the results of the test.

The MST is composed of 6 of the 18 subtests that form the McCarthy Scales of Children's Abilities (McCarthy, 1972). The subtests were chosen on the basis of content, level of difficulty, time required for administration, and ease of scoring. The subtests used include: (1) Right-Left Orientation— a measure of spatial relations, verbal concept formation, nonverbal reasoning, and directionality; (2) Verbal Memory; (3) Draw-a-Design—a measure of visual perception and visual-motor coordination; (4) Numerical Memory; (5) Conceptual Grouping—a test of logical classification skills, nonverbal reasoning, and verbal concept formation; and (6) Leg Coordination—a quick assessment of gross motor control and coordination, and balance in the child.

All tests are scored according to directions in the battery manual and good normative data are available. The MST was developed by using the standardization sample of somewhat over 100 children which was gathered for the original complete McCarthy Scales. Classification of the child is based on the criteria in the manual. Typically, the child is classified by grading each subtest as either "pass" or "fail" at a given percentile. Therefore, a general classification rule would put a child in an "at-risk" category if three or more of the tests were failed at the 30th percentile. The clinician has the option of deciding for herself the cutoff to use for any given child by using the accuracy tables provided in the manual.

All in all, the MST is a reasonably useful test battery for screening for general neuropsychological and academic dysfunction. It assesses a large number of the functional areas that should be addressed in a screening battery. Unlike the FKSB, however, the McCarthy Screening Test has not been designed to be a good statistical predictor of future difficulties and the clinician using this device is advised against using it as such.

SCREENING TEST FOR THE LURIA–NEBRASKA NEUROPSYCHOLOGICAL BATTERY

The Screening Test for the Luria–Nebraska Neuropsychological Battery (LNNB) (Golden, 1987) is not a neuropsychological screening battery per se; however, it is noted here to help clarify the purpose of the test and to help ensure that it is not used improperly by clinicians not familiar with the device. The primary purpose of the Screening Test is to predict overall performance on the age-appropriate full-length LNNB. As such the use of the test is limited to predicting which individuals will likely demonstrate "normal" or "abnormal" performance if they were administered the appropriate form of the LNNB. *The Screening Test is not designed to be used as a separate test for the diagnosis of neuropsychological deficits.*

There are two forms of the Screening Test, one for individuals ages 13 and older, and one for children between 8 and 12 years of age. Both forms of the test can easily be administered with little, if any, formal training. All of the test items for both the child and adult versions of the Screening Test come from the respective full-length LNNB. The children's form of the tests consists of 15 items, all of which can be found in the full battery. All items are scored on a zero-, one-, or two-point system with zero representing normal performance and two indicating impaired performance. Complete scoring guidelines are provided in the test manual. The items of the Screening Test are administered until the child receives a total of four or more points at which time the test is discontinued. According to the test author, if the child achieves a score of four or higher, there is a high statistical probability that administration of the complete children's version of the LNNB will reveal significant cognitive deficits. The adult version of the screening test (ages 13+) contains the same number of items with a discontinuation criterion of eight or more points. Total administration time for either version of the test is less than 20 minutes.

In general, the Screening Test for the LNNB can be useful if the clinician is interested in knowing whether to administer the complete LNNB; however, *this test should not (and cannot) be used as an indicator of cognitive dysfunction on its own.* Golden (1987) also notes that in those cases where there is a question of residual deficits from a known, past injury, or there is the question of a very mild dysfunction, the utility of the screening test is questionable, at best. (This, of course, can be considered to be the case for any individual screening test or screening battery.)

THE CLINICAL NEUROPSYCHOLOGICAL EVALUATION INSTRUMENT

The Clinical Neuropsychological Evaluation (CNE) was developed by Majovski and his colleagues (1979a, 1979b) as a clinical research device to screen for disturbances of higher cortical functions in adolescents. The CNE was based on the work of A.R. Luria and is essentially a much shortened version of a full clinical neuropsychological evaluation of the type conducted by Luria. It is comparatively brief and assesses a wide range of cognitive functions.

The CNE consists of 72 items arranged into nine functional areas: motor functions, acousticomotor organization, higher visual functions, impressive (receptive) speech, expressive speech, reading and writing, arithmetic skills, mnestic processes, and intellectual processes. The specific items can be found in the second publication (Majovski, Tanguay, Russell, Sigman, Crumley, & Goldenberg, 1979b). Each of the CNE items is scored on a four-point scale ranging from zero (no impairment) to three (severe impairment), and objective scoring criteria are provided in the original publications. Interrater reliability for the CNE ranges from 0.79 to 0.99, and thus there is support for the instrument's utility as a clinical and research tool (Goehring & Majovski, 1984).

It should be noted by the general clinician that the CNE does offer the advantages of a screening battery such as efficiency, breadth of coverage of cognitive functions, and underlying conceptual framework; however, there are a number of limitations of its validity (Majovski et al., 1979a). Above all, the CNE was not designed as a psychometric instrument, but rather, in keeping with the qualitative approach of Luria, as a *descriptive* instrument to be used for assessing possible neurological dysfunction.

An adaptation of the CNE that is more culturally appropriate to the United States, the *Children's Neuropsychological Screening Test* (CNST; Lowe, Krehbiel, Sweeney, Crumley, Peterson, Watson, & Rhodes, 1984), was designed for a slightly lower age range (approximately 8–13 years). The only published article (Lowe et al., 1984) describes the results of an initial pilot study using the CNST, which attempted to differentiate normal from at-risk learning-disabled children. The test made a discrimination between normals and special groups at a statistically significant level. This study suggests that the CNST has good potential as a screening device; however, until additional research is forthcoming, the CNST has only face validity and its conceptual underpinnings as useful feature for the clinicians. Unfortunately, the publication made no mention of the specific items used nor exactly how the CNE was adapted to create the CNST.

DISCRIMINANT EQUATION FOR SCREENING FOR NEUROPSYCHOLOGICAL ABNORMALITY

Tramontana and Boyd (1986) have reported a psychometrically based system for screening for neuropsychological abnormality in children between the ages of 8 and 16 years. The system uses a statistically derived discriminant equation (DE) that incorporates measures from the WISC-R and the Reitan–Indiana Aphasia Screening Test (AST). The WISC-R subtests used include: Information, Arithmetic, Object Assembly, Picture Completion, Similarities, and Comprehension. The AST items used are item numbers 3, 6, 9, 11, 13, 15, 16, 22a, 24, 25, 26, 30, 31, and 32. The developers of the equation note that this system capitalizes on the common use of the WISC-R and the substantial overlap that has been found between the WISC-R and other neuropsychological test results in children (Tramontana, Klee, & Boyd, 1984). The equation is as follows:

$$DE = (\text{Information} \times 0.1769) + (\text{Arithmetic} \times 0.2034) + (\text{Object Assembly} \times -0.1169) + (\text{Picture Completion} \times 0.1339) + (\text{Similarities} \times -0.1519) + (\text{Comprehension} \times 0.1661) + (\text{Dyscalculia} \times -0.8244) + (\text{Dyslexia} \times -0.8847) + (\text{Dysgraphia} \times -0.5066) + (\text{Right-Left Confusion} \times -0.5483) + (\text{Spelling Dyspraxia} \times -0.4824) - 1.6684$$

The equation is used by inserting the respective WISC-R subtest scores and either zero (absence) or one (presence) for each of the AST symptoms (see

TABLE 13-2 Symptom Categories and Scoring Criteria on the Aphasia Screening Test Used To Determine DE

Symptom categories	Item numbers
Spelling dyspraxia	3, 6, 9, 11, 24[a]
Dysgraphia	11, 21, 24
Dyslexia[b]	13, 15, 16, 22a, 30
Dyscalculia	25, 26
Right-Left confusion[c]	31, 32

[a] Spelling errors only on items 11 and 24 are included in this category. Writing errors per se (e.g., reversals, rotations, etc.) are classified under dysgraphia.
[b] Any word omission, addition, or other alteration except mispronunciation is counted as an error.
[c] Errors regarding directionality per se are included in this category. This is to be distinguished from errors resulting from failure to comprehend the task or errors involving misidentification of body parts.

Note: any error on any of the above items results in a score of 1 (presence) for the specific appropriate category.

Source: Wolf, B. A., & Tramontana, M. G. (1982). Aphasia screening test interrelationships with complete Halstead–Reitan test results for older children. *Clinical Neuropsychology, 4*, 179–186.

Table 13-2 for categories and scoring criteria). A negative number resulting from the equation predicts impairment whereas a positive number predicts nonimpairment.

The DE was derived from a sample of 90 patients who had received a comprehensive neuropsychological evaluation. In the original study, the DE yielded a 91% rate of overall correct classification. A more recent cross-validation of the utility of the equation yielded a hit rate of about 80% with a false-negative rate of 37.3% (Boyd, Tramontana, & Hooper, 1986).

In general, the DE can be a useful method of identifying those children for whom a comprehensive neuropsychological evaluation would be helpful. However, the clinician must remember that the fairly high false-negative rate may result in missing some cases, particularly those in whom the dysfunction is comparatively subtle.

14
Assessment of Very Young Children

The evaluation of the cognitive capabilities of very young children, ages 4 to 5 years and younger, presents some special problems that require a somewhat different approach to evaluation. The types of questions to be answered and the means of attempting to answer them are unique to this population. In addition to the obviously limited sample of measurable behaviors available to very young children, the influence of developmental variability discussed elsewhere in this text is particularly important when dealing with this population. Cognitive dysfunctions frequently present as diffuse disorders when commonly available measures are used. This can complicate questions concerninig diagnosis, treatment planning, and prognosis. Neurological impairment, even that which is documented through "hard data" from CT scans, EEGs, and the like, is tremendously variable in its expression from one young age to another. Even a highly circumscribed lesion in the brain may not result in the expected impairment when it occurs early in life (Fitzhugh, Fitzhugh, & Reitan, 1962).

Despite these limitations, early identification of developmental and acquired dysfunction is important. Intervention with these children during the preschool period results in greater future success for these children (Lazar & Darlington, 1978; Schweinhart & Weikart, 1980). Horton (1974) notes that even the difference between intervention initiated at age 2 versus that started at age 3 for children with impaired hearing has significant impact on subsequent language skills. In this chapter, therefore, we will discuss a few of the instruments available for use with this population. These devices will focus on global screening of a child's capabilities and will measure acquired skills in comparison to developmental norms.

GENERAL SCREENING DEVICES OF COGNITIVE ABILITIES

Denver Developmental Screening Test

The Denver Development Screening Test (DDST) (Frankenburg & Dodds, 1967; Frankenburg, Dodds, Fandel, Kazuk, & Cohrs, 1975) was designed to identify delays in development in children from birth through six years of age. The DDST was designed primarily as a screening device and its creators note that it should not be used strictly for diagnosis. Rather, significant delays in development found on the DDST should be further substantiated by using other measures such as the Bayley scales (discussed below).

The DDST measures a child's development in four specific areas: personal-social, fine motor, gross motor, and language. The personal-social section of the test assesses a child's self-help and early social skills. The fine motor section looks at the child's finger manipulation and the drawing of simple shapes. Gross motor tests assess general body control with a particular emphasis on coordination and balance. The language portion of the DDST evaluates the receptive and expressive language skills of the child.

As noted above, the DDST has been designed for screening children from birth to 6 years, although it is especially useful for screening children ages 3 months through 4 years (Gabel, Oster, & Butnik, 1986). One of the advantages of the DDST is that it is comparatively inexpensive and fairly quick and easy to administer (about 20 minutes to administer and score). No formal training in the administration of the DDST is required; however, it is a good idea for the clinician to observe a few administrations and practice on a nonclinical sample prior to the first "official" test being given.

The test is individually administered with items appropriate for the child's chronological age presented according to simple, standardized instructions. Each item is objectively scored as pass or fail. A passing response on an item indicates that the child is able to perform the tested behavior which is defined as a skill demonstrated by 90% of the normative group younger than the child. Total test results are then determined to be "normal," "questionable," or "abnormal" according to the number of failed or untestable items within the four sections of the test.

The clinician should be aware that there is research that indicates that the DDST does not consistently identify preschool and primary students with significant neurological and/or neurodevelopmental disorders (Sterling & Sterling, 1977). In addition, the standardization sample for the DDST has been criticized as underrepresenting some socioeconomic groups (Werner, 1972).

Developmental Screening Inventory

The Developmental Screening Inventory (DSI; Gesell & Amatruda, 1947) was designed to establish a child's current developmental status and screen for the presence of delays in development. The test was based on the developmental schedules created by Gesell and his associates (1949).

The DSI assesses development in five major categories: adaptive skills (sensorimotor and problem-solving antecedents of intelligence), gross motor, fine motor, language, and personal-social. Representative items from each section appear at discrete age levels through the scale—at 4-week intervals through 1 year of age, at 3-month intervals from 1 to 2 years, and at 6-month intervals to age 3 years. The placement of items was determined through research so that 50% of infants identified as normal would pass at the given age level. Although administration of the DSI requires no formal training, the clinician should be experienced in working with infants and very young children and should be thoroughly familiar with the DSI materials and manual.

The DSI administration requires a flat surface on which the child can demonstrate motor behaviors, a table for object manipulation, and the following test objects which must be provided by the clinician: an embroidery hoop, a small cup, 10 one-inch wooden cubes, crayon, book, and a small toy. Items are scored as pass or fail and are judged from behaviors observed during the course of the evaluation, behaviors elicited by the presentation of test objects, and/or a developmental history obtained from the child's parent(s) or primary care-giver. Administration procedures and scoring rules and criteria are clearly presented in the test manual. Testing begins at the child's chronological age and continues in each developmental area until she is unable to pass any items at two consecutive age levels.

Although Gesell's original intention was that his technique be used as a guide for clinical evaluation with qualitative descriptions taking precedence over numerical values, a developmental quotient can be calculated for each of the areas of development assessed in the test. A developmental quotient of less than 70 in any area suggests abnormal functioning in that domain and the need for more thorough evaluation.

Slosson Intelligence Test

The Slosson Intelligence Test is a brief individual test of intelligence designed to provide screening information on individuals from infancy through adulthood (Slosson, 1963). The test assesses mental ages from 2 weeks through 26 years. Test questions in the Slosson emphasize mathematical reasoning, vocabulary, auditory memory, and general information. The primary advantages of the Slosson are its relative ease and quickness of administration and the objective scoring system (Hunt, 1972).

The Slosson test questions are presented to the child sequentially in ascending difficulty with each question labeled according to the age level that the average child should be able to pass. Although the test is comprised of 194 items, the examiner will usually administer far less to the child because of the basal and ceiling levels that are established as the test progresses (Gabel et al., 1986). Most questions require a verbal response from the child except for eight items in which geometric figures must be reproduced, and in the infant portion, where postural control and locomotion are assessed.

Scoring is expressed in age-months and credit is given by $\frac{1}{2}$ month credits during year 1, 1-month credits during years 2 to 4, by 2-month credits during years 5 to 15, and by 3-month credits during years 16–26. Both a mental age and an estimated IQ score can be derived from the data obtained during testing.

The Slosson has received a good deal of criticism on a number of key points. The manner of IQ estimate calculation is a serious drawback to the test in that the standard deviations differ greatly throughout the age ranges of the test which significantly limits comparisons across ages (Gabel et al., 1986). The Slosson places an inordinate emphasis on verbal skills, making the test less useful for children ages 2 to 3, particularly if language has been delayed or middle-class language patterns are not a part of the child's environment (Hunt, 1972). At the earliest levels of the test, behaviors are not well represented due to a small sample of test items (Sattler, 1982). The test manual does not include demographic data for the standardization group and the standardization sample appears only to have been drawn from the New York state region (Himelstein, 1972). Because of such serious limitations, the use of the Slosson is not advised except in those circumstances where time is extremely limited and major educational (or other significant) decisions are not to be made on the basis of test results.

Bayley Scales of Infant Development

The Bayley Scales of Infant Development are a well-standardized measure of development in infants and young children from ages 2 months to $2\frac{1}{2}$ years (Bayley, 1969). These scales are generally considered to be the instrument of choice for the assessment of infant and very young child development (Gabel et al., 1986; Hartlage & Telzrow, 1986). The reliability and validity of the test has been well established (Gabel et al., 1986) and it provides valuable information about early mental and motor development as well as establishing the presence of developmental delays. An initial administration of the Bayley scales for a specific child can provide a baseline against which later evaluations can be compared to determine rates of cognitive growth and development.

There are three separate scales that make up the Bayley: a Mental scale, a Motor scale, and an Infant Behavior Record. The Mental Scale consists of 163 items arranged in chronological order beginning at the 2 month level and ending at the 30-month level. In the earliest months, the Mental Scale assesses sensory integrity and efficiency including visual fixation and tracking, and auditory awareness and localization. Later in the scale, more complex cognitive activities and processes are evaluated such as purposeful manipulation of objects, visual discrimination, early language development, and memory.

Eighty-one items make up the Motor scale which assesses both fine and gross motor abilities. Each mental and motor scale item is numbered and assigned two age markers: one for the average age at which an item is passed and a range in which 95% of the standardization sample passed the item. The age range is useful in clarifying the individual variability seen in normal child development.

The Mental Scale yields a Mental Development Index and the Motor Scale yields a Psychomotor Development Index, both of which have means of 100 and standard deviations of 16. The resulting standard scores can be interpreted similarly to standard IQ scores in the sense that deficient performance is considered to be that which occurs two or more standard deviations below the mean. Bayley scale scores *cannot* to equated to IQ scores.

The Infant Behavior Record, which is not a formal test, per se, is administered during the evaluation. Rather, it is a systematic method for observing, recording, and assessing several key behavioral and emotional features that may occur during the examination. Ratings concerning 11 areas (social orientation, cooperation, fearfulness, tension, emotional tone, object orientation, goal directedness, attention span, endurance, activity, and reactivity) can be compared to the normative data provided in the test manual. The resulting record of behavior essentially helps to objectify behavioral observations.

Unlike many of the test instruments described in this chapter and elsewhere in the book, the Bayley scales require that the examiner be thoroughly trained in the administration and observation techniques. The clinician should be very comfortable with and accustomed to being with infants and should be well versed in normal patterns of development. The average administration time for the test is about 45 minutes. Although it is preferable for the clinician to see the child alone, it may be necessary to have the child's parent with her in the testing room to increase the likelihood of maximal cooperation.

Common administration problems include the failure to develop an adequate rapport with the child and an inability to keep the child sufficiently interested in the tasks at hand to complete the entire examination. With increased experience in the administration of the Bayley, such problems frequently diminish to a large extent, however.

Stanford–Binet Intelligence Scale

The Stanford–Binet Intelligence Scale, now in its fourth edition (Thorndike, Hagen, & Sattler, 1986), is one of the oldest and most widely used instruments for the measurement of general intelligence in young children. In its current edition, the test provides a general measure of intellectual functioning in children from 2 years of age through adulthood. Test items are ordered chronologically in discrete age groupings under the assumption, dating back to the original version of the test, that an average child should be able to pass all of the tests through her own chronological age grouping. From ages 2 to 6 years, test items are grouped at six-month intervals. At age 6 years and upwards, test items are grouped at yearly intervals. Each age level has six tests as well as a supplemental test in the event that one of the tests was invalidated because of administration errors. Between 2 and 6 years of age each passed test receives 1 month of credit whereas from 6 years of age and on, each test passed received 2 months of credit.

The Stanford–Binet test items assess a variety of diverse verbal and nonverbal functions including receptive and expressive language, short-term visual and auditory memory, verbal and nonverbal reasoning, and visual-spatial organization. Unfortunately, the test has been designed such that specific functioning in a particular area of cognitive abilities is difficult to assess since the different abilities tested occur unevenly throughout the scale. For instance, assessment of verbal abilities is extremely limited in the early parts of the Stanford–Binet while visual-spatial functions seem to be emphasized, and the reverse is true at the older age levels. Thus, as a comprehensive screening device, the Stanford–Binet does have its limitations unless the child to be evaluated is within a very limited age range (roughly 4–7 years) where verbal and nonverbal abilities are assessed almost equally.

A number of criticisms have been raised about the utility of earlier versions of the test (Gabel et al., 1986) including a heavy reliance on verbal responding at all age levels and the aforementioned uneven distribution of test items for specific abilities. These difficulties have called into question the utility of the Stanford–Binet for education treatment planning (Helton, Workman, & Matuzek, 1982) and have resulted in a widespread acceptance of different measures of intelligence such as the various child versions of the Wechsler scales. Proponents of the most recent revision of the test note that many of the earlier criticisms have been addressed (Thorndike et al, 1986). The newest version of the Stanford–Binet appears to be a significant improvement over the older forms of the test; however, it will take time for the necessary research to be conducted to validate the clinical utility of the latest version.

Leiter International Performance Scale

There are occasions when a clinician is asked to assess the functioning of a young child who is nonverbal, has been severely culturally deprived, or has limited language skills. In such instances, the Leiter International Performance Scale (Leiter, 1948) can be useful. It was designed to be used with children ranging in age from 3 to 18 years. The Leiter's primary use is for estimating intellectual functioning in individuals who cannot be evaluated with more conventional measures such as the Wechsler scales or Stanford–Binet. Such individuals would include those with hearing, speech, or other types of language handicaps. It is also useful in the assessment of those children with motor handicaps.

The Leiter consists of a slotted wooden frame that accepts a different cardboard template for each of the various tests that comprise the total scale. Each test is comprised of a number of wooden blocks that can be arranged to fit into the frame to complete a theme or solve a problem based on that which is depicted on the cardboard template. The Leiter makes use of the concept of mental age. There are 54 standardized tests within the scale that involve activities such as color matching, analogies, series completion, visual discrimination, and block construction. There are six tests within each of the age groupings that appear at yearly intervals from ages 2 through 18 years. As the testing proceeds, a basal level of performance is established at which all tests are passed, and proceeds up to a test performance ceiling, which is the first age group at which all tests are failed.

Since the Leiter's primary use is with children who are hearing or speech impaired, the standardized administration makes use of nonverbal instructions. In most cases, the examiner either points to the materials in a prescribed manner or completes a portion of the subtest to demonstrate the problem-solving strategy to be used for the subtest. The child is usually started well below her chronological age so that she has the opportunity to fully understand the general problem-solving expectations that underlie the test. Average administration time for the scale is 30–45 minutes.

Although there have been many limitations of the test noted (e.g., Sattler, 1982), the most significant of which are its outdated normative data and inadequate standardization by today's standards, the Leiter Scale continues to be used with those children who, because of their impairments, cannot be tested with more traditional psychometric devices.

SCREENING FOR SOCIAL AND ADAPTIVE BEHAVIOR

Very young children often are not cooperative in a testing situation for a variety of reasons. In addition, the assessment devices briefly discussed above sometimes do not offer enough information to make definitive statements concerning the infant's or young child's cognitive status. Cognitive deficits often are reflected in a young child's adaptive and social behaviors (Hartlage & Telzrow, 1986). Thus, the clinician periodically may need to supplement her test data for a child, and the use of adaptive behavior scales is an effective approach. As a general rule, it is a good idea for such a procedure to be performed as a matter of course when evaluating a young child as these measures establish a good baseline from which to make comparisons as the child continues to develop.

American Association on Mental Deficiency Adaptive Behavior Scale

The American Association on Mental Deficiency (AAMD) Adaptive Behavior Scale (ABS) is a behavior rating scale that assesses the child's behavioral and adaptive competencies in developmentally disabled, mentally retarded, and emotionally disturbed individuals (Nihira, Foster, Shellhaas, & Leland, 1974). The scale contains two parts. The first portion consists of those behavioral domains and survival skills considered as necessary for independent daily living. The behavioral domains include independent functioning (e.g., eating, appearance, personal hygiene), physical development, economic activity, numbers and time, language development, domestic activity, self-direction, responsibility, and socialization.

The second portion of the ABS focuses on maladaptive behaviors. It includes 14 behaviors related to personality and behavior disorders. These behaviors include: violent/destructive behaviors, antisocial behavior, rebellious behavior, untrustworthy behavior, withdrawal, stereotyped behavior or odd mannerisms, inappropriate interpersonal behaviors, unacceptable vocal habits, unacceptable or eccentric habits, self-abusive behaviors, hyperactive tendencies, sexually aberrant behavior, psychological disorders, and the use of medications.

The ABS can be easily administered by examiners or clinicians with little formal training in the procedures. Scoring is simple and objective with an average administration time of 15–30 minutes. The examiner goes through the items with a person familiar enough with the child to make the necessary ratings. The informant can be a parent, care-giver, etc. Raw scores obtained for both parts of the scale are converted into percentile-referenced standard scores. The test manual provides scores for 11 age groups ranging from 3 to 69 years of age. Treatment planning is based on the child's strengths and weaknesses.

A version of the scale was restandardized in 1975 for use in public schools—the AAMB-ABS Public School Version which can be used with children from 7 years, 3 months to 13 years, 2 months (Lambert, Windmiller, Cole, & Figueroa, 1975). This version of the ABS is identical to the original except for the elimination of some domains not applicable to school settings. Administration procedures are basically the same, with parents and teachers being the primary informants. The revised version of the ABS has been described as useful for profiling adaptive behavior strengths and weaknesses, and developing intervention plans for a child (Sattler, 1982).

The Vineland Scales

The Vineland Social Maturity Scale (Doll, 1935) is the best known and probably the most widely used measure of social competence. It was designed to measure self-help skills, self-direction, and responsibility in individuals from birth through adulthood. The scale was first published in 1935 with numerous revisions occurring through 1965. In 1984, the scales were completely restructured, reconceptualized, restandardized, and renamed—*The Vineland Adaptive* Behavior Scales (Sparrow, Balla, & Cicchetti, 1984).

Although the Vineland is not an intelligence test, it can be used to obtain developmental data when a child is unresponsive, uncooperative, or unavailable for direct assessment (Gabel et al, 1986). The administration of the test requires a trained examiner who is familiar with the scale items and interview procedures. It takes roughly 20–30 minutes to administer the Vineland and the child's parent or major caretaker is usually the informant. In a structured interview format, the examiner determines how the child typically performs the particular behavior in question. A "pass" for a behavior is given only if the child usually performs a behavior, not if the child is capable of the behavior but typically does not engage in it. The interview proceeds from one category of behavior to another and a basal and ceiling score are established in each category. The categories of behavior assessed in the older version of the Vineland (Social Maturity Scale) are presented in Table 14-1.

TABLE 14-1 Categories of Behavior Assessed by the Vineland Social Maturity Scale

Category	Types of behavior assessed
Self-help–General	Early physical maturation, mobility, toileting, telling time
Self-help–Eating	Mechanics of eating (e.g., drinking from a cup unassisted, cares for self at table, etc.)
Self-help–Dressing	Dressing and bathing skills
Locomotion	Directed movement (e.g., crawling, travels unassisted around town, etc.)
Occupation	Productive use of time
Communication	Conveying and receiving information
Self-direction	Taking financial and personal responsibility
Socialization	Assessment of relationships with others

The Vineland (revised version) now has three distinct scales that can be used in differing circumstances: two interview scales (one brief scale and a longer one suited for institutional programming purposes) and a checklist form for use by teachers. These scales assess adaptive functioning in individuals from birth through 19 years of age. The teacher scale was designed for use with children 3 to 13 years. Adaptive function is assessed in five domains and subdomains (Table 14-2). The classroom scale evaluates the first four of these domains. The preliminary work done with the new Vineland scales indicate that they are clinically useful (Gabel et al., 1986).

TABLE 14-2 Domains of Behavior Assessed by the Vineland Adaptive Behavior Scale

Domain	Subdomain
Communication	Receptive language Expressive language Written language
Daily living skills	Personal Domestic Community
Socialization	Interpersonal relationships Play and leisure time Coping skills
Motor skills	Gross motor skills Fine motor skills
Maladaptive behavior	None

Appendices

Appendix A: Sample Interview Form

This questionnaire is meant to be administered orally. The clinician can follow up any questions with a more in-depth assessment if the informant's answers indicate any problems.

Date _____

I. Background Information
Child's name _____ (Nickname) _____
Birth date _____ Age _____
Referral source _____
Reason for referral (given by referral source)
_____

Parents' names _____
Informant for interview _____
Child's address _____ Telephone _____
_____

Name of school _____
Names and ages of siblings (indicate whether half-, step-, or full-sibling)
_____
_____

Name of pediatrician _____
Names and specialties of other professionals who have treated the child
_____
_____

II. Presenting Problem (in the informant's words)
_____
_____
_____

III. Prenatal History
Was the child adopted? (If so, is the information from records or from interview with the biological mother?) _____
List any pregnancy complications and the month of pregnancy during which they occurred. (Examples: anemia, high blood pressure, swollen ankles

[mother's], German measles, toxemia, Rh incompatibility, any diseases of the mother)

_____
_____
_____

Did the mother have any hospitalizations or surgeries during pregnancy? If so, state the reason.

_____
_____

Did the mother experience any severe shock or emotional strain during pregnancy? If so, describe.

_____

What medications, prescription and otherwise, were taken during pregnancy?

_____

Did the mother smoke during pregnancy? If so, what was the amount?
_____

Did the mother drink alcohol during pregnancy? If so, how much?
_____

List all other pregnancies, including miscarriages and abortions. State the times and reasons for miscarriages.

_____
_____

IV. Natal and Perinatal History
Name of hospital where the child was delivered _____
List medications given to mother during birth _____

Length of time for labor _____
List anesthesias used during birth _____
Was labor induced? Why? _____
Was the child delivered head first? _____
Was there use of forceps or a cesarean section? _____
Was the baby born with any bruises or unusual birthmarks? _____
Were there any unusual circumstances of the birth? (Examples: umbilical cord wrapped around the baby's neck, breathing problems, unusual color of skin) Describe. _____

_____
_____

Appendix A

Did the infant receive any special medical treatment? (Examples: blood transfusions, oxygen, medications, use of incubator) _____

V. Early Development
Were there any feeding problems? Describe. (Examples: colic, special feeding formula) _____

Was the infant breast fed? How long? _____
Any unusual sleeping patterns? Describe. _____
At what age did the child:
First sit without support? _____
Stand without support? _____
Walk? _____
Babble and coo? _____
Put together words meaningfully? _____
Talk in complete sentences? _____
Become toilet trained? _____
Stop wetting the bed? _____
Did the child cry excessively? _____
Was the child unusually quiet? _____
(The clinician should obtain a more complete developmental history if any unusual patterns are reported.)
Were there any unusual growth patterns (height or weight)? Describe.
_____
_____

VI. Social Development
At what age did the child begin to play independently with other children?
_____

What is the quality of interactions with siblings? _____

What are the names and ages of children with whom the child plays regularly? _____

In what activities does the child engage with these friends? _____

VII. Academic History
At what age did the child begin school? _____
Current grade level. _____
Were any grades repeated? State reason. _____
Have there been any changes in the child's grades or teacher evaluations?
_____

(The clinician should contact school personnel for corroboration.)

VIII. Medical History

Have there been any previous evaluations of the child? State dates, reasons, and names of the professionals involved. _____
_____

State the diseases and illnesses experienced by the child. Include dates and treatment, if any. _____
_____

State the medications that the child is currently taking. _____

List the surgeries experienced by the child. Include dates, reasons, and length of hospitalizations. _____

Was the child hospitalized for any other reasons? State dates, lengths, reasons, and treatments received. _____

Has the child ever had high fevers? Did the child experience convulsions as a result? State dates and treatments. _____
_____

Has the child ever had fainting spells? Was treatment given? _____
_____

Has the child ever been evaluated for hearing difficulties, speech problems, or vision problems? State dates and treatments. _____
_____

Does the child have any allergies? State date diagnosed and treatment given.
Has the child ever sustained a head injury? _____
Did the child lose consciousness? If so, for how long? _____
____

What medical treatment was given for the injury? _____
_____

Has the child ever had seizures (convulsions, epileptic fits)? What treatment was given? _____
_____

IX. Behavioral and Emotional Functioning

(The clinician may want to use a structured assessment as well.)
How would you describe your child's personality? _____
_____

What are the child's favorite toys and games? _____
_____

Does the child play well with others? _____
Is the child moody? _____

Appendix A

How does the child respond to frustration? _____
How does the child show displeasure? _____
How does the child show happiness? _____
What are the child's chores and responsibilities? _____

_____

What forms of discipline are used with the child and what are the effects of these methods? _____

_____
_____

X. Family

Who lives with the child? What are their relationships to the child?

_____
_____

Are the parents separated or divorced? _____
What languages are spoken in the home? _____
Have the child's siblings had any medical illnesses or behavioral problems? Describe them. _____

_____

Did either of the parents have childhood medical conditions, behavioral problems, or emotional problems? Describe. _____

_____

Have any close relatives had any of the following disorders?
Neurological disease _____
Academic problems _____
Epilepsy _____
Visual problems _____
Hearing problems _____
Speech problems _____
Delayed development _____
Learning problems _____
Emotional problems _____
Is there anything else you feel might be important in understanding your child's problems? _____

_____
_____

Appendix B: Common Tests Used in the Assessment of School-Aged Children

TEST	PUBLISHER
COGNITIVE FUNCTIONS	
Wechsler Intelligence Scale for Children-Revised (WISC-R)	The Psychological Corporation
Kaufman Assessment Battery for Children (K-ABC)	American Guidance Service
Stanford–Binet Intelligence Scale	Riverside Publishing Company
Leiter International Performance Scale	Stoelting Publishing Company
Woodcock–Johnson Psychoeducational Battery (WJPB)-Cognitive Scale	DLM-Teaching Resources
BASIC LANGUAGE FUNCTIONS—Listening and Speaking	
Test of Language Development-Primary (TOLD-P)	PRO-ED
Test of Language Development-Intermediate (TOLD-I)	PRO-ED
Test of Adolescent Language (TOAL)	PRO-ED
Clinical Evaluation of Language Functions (CELF)	Charles Merrill
Token Test for Children	DLM-Teaching Resources
Diagnostic Achievement Battery	PRO-ED
Aphasia Screening Test	Neuropsychology Press
Boehm Test of Basic Concepts	The Psychological Corporation
READING	
Woodcock Test of Reading Mastery	American Guidance Service
K-ABC Achievement Scale	American Guidance Service
Woodcock–Johnson Psychoeducational (WJPB)-Achievement Scale	DLM-Teaching Resources
Diagnostic Reading Scales	CTB/McGraw Hill
Diagnostic Achievement Battery	PRO-ED
Boder Test of Reading-Spelling Patterns	Grune & Stratton, Inc.
Kaufman Tests of Educational Achievement	American Guidance Service

Appendix B

WRITING

Woodcock–Johnson Psychoeducational (WJPB)-Achievement Scale	DLM-Teaching Resources
Test of Written Language (TOWL)	PRO-ED
Test of Adolescent Language (TOAL)	PRO-ED
Aphasia Screening Test	Neuropsychology Press
Diagnostic Achievement Battery	PRO-ED
Kaufman Tests of Educational Achievement	American Guidance Service

ARITHMETIC

K-ABC Achievement Battery	American Guidance Service
Woodcock–Johnson Psychoeducational (WJPB)-Achievement Scale	DLM-Teaching Resources
Key Math Test	American Guidance Service
Kaufman Tests of Educational Achievement	American Guidance Service

MOTOR/VISUAL-MOTOR FUNCTIONING

Finger Tapping	Reitan Neuropsychology Laboratory
Grip Strength	Reitan Neuropsychology Laboratory
Aphasia Screening Test	Neuropsychology Press
Developmental Test of Visual Motor Integration (Beery VMI)	Follett Publishing Company
Bender Visual-Motor Gestalt Test	The Psychological Corporation
Physical Dexterity Tests-System of Multi-Cultural Pluralistic Assessment (SOMPA)	The Psychological Corporation

SENSORY FUNCTIONING

Sensory-Perceptual Examination	Neuropsychology Press
Sensory-Perceptual Tasks	See Benton, Hamsher, Varney, & Spreen, 1983; Reitan, 1979
Motor Free Visual Perception Test	The Psychological Corporation

MEMORY FUNCTIONS

Digit Span Tests	
WISC-R	The Psychological Corporation
K-ABC	American Guidance Service
Stanford–Binet Intelligence Test	Riverside Publishing Company
ITPA	Western Psychological Services
Rey Auditory Verbal Learning	See Rey, 1964
Wechsler Memory Scale-Revised	The Psychological Corporation
McCarthy Scales Verbal Memory	The Psychological Corporation
Selective and Restricted Reminding	See Buschke, 1974a, 1974b; Buschke & Fuld, 1974; Hannay & Levin, 1985
Benton Visual Retention Test	The Psychological Corporation
Rey–Osterrieth Complex Figure	See Rey, 1941; Osterrieth, 1944
Tactual Performance Test	Reitan Neuropsychology Laboratory
The Knox Cube Test	See Sterne, 1966

SOCIAL BEHAVIOR

Connors Behavior Rating Scale	(See Connors, 1969; 1982)
Child Behavior Checklist	University Associates in Psychiatry
Vineland Social Maturity Scales	American Guidance Service

COMPLEX PROBLEM-SOLVING

Trail Making Test	Reitan Neuropsychology Laboratory
Halstead Category Test	Reitan Neuropsychology Laboratory

SYMPTOM CHECKLISTS

Neuropsychological Status Examination	Psychological Assessment Resources
Neuropsychological Symptom Checklist	Psychological Assessment Resources

Adapted from: Hartlage, L. C., & Telzrow, C. F. (1986). *Neuropsychological assessment and intervention with children and adolescents.* Sarasota, Florida: Professional Resource Exchange. Adapted with permission.

Appendix C: Common Tests Used in the Assessment of Preschool-Aged Children

TEST	PUBLISHER
COGNITIVE FUNCTIONS	
Wechsler Preschool and Primary Scale of Intelligence (WPPSI)	The Psychological Corporation
Kaufman Assessment Battery for Children (K-ABC)	American Guidance Service
Stanford–Binet Intelligence Scale	Riverside Publishing Company
Leiter International Performance Scale	Stoelting Publishing Company
Woodcock–Johnson Psychoeducational Battery (WJPB)-Cognitive Scale	DLM-Teaching Resources
McCarthy Scales of Children's Abilities	The Psychological Corporation
Bayley Scales of Infant Development	The Psychological Corporation
Hiskey–Nebraska Test of Learning Aptitude	Author
BASIC LANGUAGE FUNCTIONS	
Receptive-Expressive Language Scale (REEL)	University Park Press
Test of Early Language Development (TELD)	DLM-Teaching Resources
Clinical Evaluation of Language Functions (CELF)	Charles Merrill
Token Test for Children	DLM-Teaching Resources
Preschool Language Scale	Charles Merrill
Language Sample of 50 Utterances	Charles Merrill
Peabody Picture Vocabulary Test-Revised (PPVT-R)	American Guidance Service
Expressive One Word Picture	American Guidance Service
K-ABC Achievement	American Guidance Service
Test for Auditory Comprehension of Language (TACL)	DLM-Teaching Resources
Boehm Test of Basic Concepts	The Psychological Corporation
Goldman–Fristoe–Woodcock Auditory Skills Battery	American Guidance Service
Illinois Test of Psycholinguistic Abilities	Western Psychological Services

PRE-ACADEMIC SKILLS

K-ABC Achievement Scales	American Guidance Service
WJPB Achievement Scales	DLM-Teaching Resources

MOTOR FUNCTIONING

Finger Tapping (age 5+)	Reitan Neuropsychology Laboratory
Grip Strength (age 5+)	Reitan Neuropsychology Laboratory
Developmental Test of Visual Motor Integration (Beery VMI)	Follett Publishing Company
Bender Visual-Motor Gestalt Test	The Psychological Corporation
Bayley Scales of Infant Development	The Psychological Corporation
Bruinks–Oseretsky Tests of Motor Proficiency	American Guidance Service
Purdue Pegboard	Lafayette Instrument Company

SENSORY FUNCTIONING

Sensory-Perceptual Examination (age 5+)	Neuropsychology Press
Sensory Perceptual Tasks	(See Benton, Hamsher, Varney & Spreen, 1983; Reitan, 1979)
Motor Free Visual Perception Test	The Psychological Corporation

MEMORY FUNCTIONS

Digit Span Tests	The Psychological Corporation
WPPSI	
K-ABC	American Guidance Service
Stanford–Binet Intelligence Test	Riverside Publishing Company
ITPA	Western Psychological Services
WPPSI Sentences Test	The Psychological Corporation
Rey Auditory Verbal Learning	See Rey, 1964
McCarthy Scales Verbal Memory	The Psychological Corporation
The Knox Cube Test	See Sterne, 1966 Also, Stoelting Publishing Company

SOCIAL BEHAVIOR

Child Behavior Checklist	University Associates in Psychiatry
Vineland Social Maturity Scales	American Guidance Service
Carey Infant Temperament Scale	Author
California Preschool Social Competency Scale	Consulting Psychologists Press

DEVELOPMENTAL INVENTORIES

Vineland Social Maturity Scales	American Guidance Service
Minnesota Child Development Inventory (MCDI)	Behavior Science Systems
Developmental Profile II	Psychological Developmental Publications
Battelle Developmental Inventory	DLM-Teaching Resources

Adapted from: Hartlage, L. C., & Telzrow, C. F. (1986). *Neuropsychological assessment and intervention with children and adolescents.* Sarasota, Florida: Professional Resource Exchange. Adapted with permission.

Appendix D: Test Publisher Addresses

Academic Therapy Publications
20 Commercial Boulevard
Novato, California 94947-6191

American Guidance Services
Publishers' Building
Circle Pines, Minnesota 55014-1796

Behavior Science Systems
P.O. Box 1108
Minneapolis, Minnesota 55440

Consulting Psychologists Press, Inc.
577 College Avenue
Palo Alto, California 94306

CTB McGraw-Hill
Del Monte Research Park
Monterey, California 93940

Devereux Foundation Press
19 South Waterloo Road
Devon, Pennsylvania 19333

DLM-Teaching Resources
One DLM Park
Allen, Texas 75002

Follett Publishing Company
4506 Northwest Highway
Crystal Lake, Illinois 60014

Grune & Stratton, Inc.
111 Fifth Avenue
New York, New York 10003

Lafayette Instrument Company
P.O. Box 5729
Sagamore Parkway
Lafayette, Indiana 47903

Marshall S. Hiskey
5640 Baldwin
Lincoln, Nebraska

Charles E. Merrill Publishing Company
1300 Alum Creek Drive
Box 508
Columbus, Ohio 43216

Neuropsychology Press
1338 East Edison Street
Tucson, Arizona 85719

PRO-ED
5341 Industrial Oaks Boulevard
Austin, Texas 78735

Psychological Assessment Resources, Inc.
P.O. Box 998
Odessa, Florida 33556

The Psychological Corporation
555 Academic Court
San Antonio, Texas 78204

Psychological Development Publications
P.O. Box 3198
Aspen, Colorado 81612

Reitan Neuropsychology Laboratory
1338 East Edison Avenue
Tucson, Arizona 87519

The Riverside Publishing Company
8420 Bryn Mawr Avenue
Chicago, Illinois 60631

Stoelting Company
1350 South Kostner Avenue
Chicago, Illinois 60623

University Associates in Psychiatry
One South Prospect Street
Burlington, Vermont 05401

University Park Press
233 East Redwood Street
Baltimore, Maryland 21203

Western Psychological Services
12031 Wilshire Boulevard
Los Angeles, California 90025

Glossary

abducens nerve—The VIth cranial nerve. Lesions here can result in excessive lacrimation.
abscess—A circumscribed infection characterized by a build up of pus surrounded by a thick wall of cells.
absence seizures—A form of epilepsy, frequently found in children, characterized by a brief altered state of consciousness. Also known as petit mal seizures.
abulia—Inability to perform voluntary acts or make decisions.
acalculia—Sometimes called dyscalculia, this is an acquired reduction in the ability of a person to perform arithmetic calculations.
achromatopsia—Loss of color vision. It is usually associated with an infarct in the distribution of the posterior cerebral artery, but it is also possible from other lesions involving ventromedial occipital lesions where it is limited to the contralateral hemifield.
acoustic nerve—The VIIIth cranial nerve. It has two divisions, the cochlear division which is partly responsible for the transmission of auditory information to the brain, and the vestibular division which is responsible for the sense of balance.
acoustic neuroma—A tumor, largely composed of nerve cells and nerve fibers, that often compromises function of the acoustic division of the VIIIth cranial nerve.
acromegaly—A chronic disease of the endocrine system resulting in elongation and enlargement of certain bone structures, including the frontal bones and jaw bones. Symptoms include muscular pain, headaches, and sweating.
Addison's disease—A condition resulting from a deficiency in secretion of adrenocortical hormones. Symtoms include anorexia, weight loss, nausea, weakness, and fatigue.
afferent fibers—Neuronal pathways that carry information upward toward the cerebral cortex from peripheral areas of the nervous system.

agnosia—Literally, a condition of not knowing. It is the inability to recognize sensory stimuli. Color agnosia is the inability to recognize colors. Visual agnosia is the inability to recognize objects in the presence of intact visual sensation.

agrammatism—A defect in the syntactical compostion of the patient's verbal output . It is characterized by the omission of most relational words including articles, prepositions, and conjunctions.

agraphia—An acquired condition of impaired or absent writing ability.

agyria—A condition marked by relative absence of the gyral convolutions of the cortex. It results from abnormal migration of neural cells during gestation.

akathisia—A condition of extreme motor restlessness. It is accompanied by subjective feelings of anxiety and restlessness.

akinesia—A state of lowered motor activity.

akinetic mutism—A state of wakeful unresponsiveness in which there is no apparent purposeful mental activity. The person appears to be awake, but inactive.

alexia—An acquired inability to read.

amnesia—A partial or total impairment of the memory functions. Anterograde amnesia is a disturbance of memory that follows some etiological event. It is disturbance of the transfer of engrams from short-term into long-term memory storage. Retrograde amnesia is a disturbance of memory prior to the etiological event. It is a disturbance of retrieval from long-term storage.

amygdala—One of the structures of the limbic system, important in memory and in the regulation of emotion.

amyotrophic lateral sclerosis—A condition of muscle weakness and atrophy with spasticity and hyperreflexia. It is the result of degeneration of motor neurons of the spinal cord, medulla, and cortex.

anencephaly—A congenital condition in which the child is born missing most of the forebrain as well as parts of the brain stem and cerebellum. It is probably due to exposure to neurotoxic or cytotoxic chemicals during the first month of pregnancy, resulting in a failure of the anterior neural tube to close. Frequently the infant is miscarried or stillborn.

aneurysm—A weak wall of a vein or artery that dilates and fills with blood and that may hemorrhage, destoying surrounding neural tissue.

angular gyrus—A region of the cerebral cortex, in the area of the posterior parietal lobe, that is intimately involved in the production of speech.

anisocoria—A condition where in the pupils dilate unevenly to light.

anomia—Sometimes known as dysnomia, it is a condition in which the patient has difficulty finding the correct word. It is often assessed by a confrontation naming task.

anosmia—Lack of the sense of smell. Although it is sometimes associated with lesions in the olfactory nerve (cranial nerve I), it is more frequently associated with non-central nervous system dysfunction such as peripheral disease of the nostrils.

anosognosia—A condition in which the patient is unaware of her deficits. It occurs despite objective evidence that such a deficit exists and is often associated with lesions in the nondominant hemisphere.

anterior cerebral artery—An artery that originates from the internal carotid artery and principally serves the frontal lobes, corpus callosum, and olfactory and optic tracts.

anterior communicating artery—An artery that originates from the anterior cerebral artery, supplies the caudate nucleus, and forms part of the Circle of Willis.

anterograde amnesia—Loss of memory for events that occurred following cerebral trauma, such as often occurs in head injuries.

anticholinergic drugs—Drugs that interfere with passage of nerve impulses through the parasympathetic fibers.

Anton's syndrome—A form of anosognosia in which the patient is totally blind but lacks awareness of his blindness.

aphasia—An acquired inability to use certain aspects of language. Aphasia can be either an expressive or a receptive language disorder. Aphasia is a very broad term which is made more useful by descriptive qualifiers to indicate the type of language impairment involved.

aphemia—Nonfluent speech with intact writing skills.

apraxia—Impaired ability to perform previously chained skills in a continuous behavior. Construction apraxia is an impairment in reproducing patterns which is assessed by drawing and drafting or by having the patient build three-demensional objects. Ideational apraxia is impairment in the idea of the required behavior and is usually assessed by asking the patient to perform several linked behaviors. Ideomotor apraxia is the inability to demonstrate motor behaviors that were known in the past and is assessed by asking the patient to pantomime a task such as using a can opener or using a pair of scissors.

aprosody—A condition in which the coloring, rhythm, melody, cadence, intonation, or emphasis of speech is impaired. A person with this condition is likely to speak in a monotone despite relaying affective material.

Aqueduct of Sylvius—A narrow canal, about three-quarters of an inch long, that connects that third and fourth ventricles.

arachnoid—The middle layer of the meninges. The term means "like a spiderweb" and is used because of the delicate nature of the arachnoid.

arachnoid space—The space around the arachnoid layer that is filled with fibrous tissue and acts as a conduit for cerebrospinal fluid.

astereognosis—An acquired inability to recognize an object by the sense of touch. It is assessed by handing an object to a blindfolded patient and asking the patient to identify the object.

astrocytoma—A type of neoplasm that develops form astrocyte cells. These tumors are typically unencapsulated and intracerebral.

ataxia—Loss or failure of muscular coordination. Movement, especially gait, which is clumsy and appears to be uncertain. The patient may sway while walking. Ataxia usually results from an inaccurate sense of position caused by distorted proprioception in the lower limbs. The problems increase greatly when the patient is asked to walk with eyes closed.

athetosis—A type of movement disorder in which involuntary undulating, or writhing movements are made slowly. (These are called athetoid movements.) They are slower and more sustained than choreiform movements and are associated with increased muscle tone.

atonia—Complete lack of muscle tone.

atrophy—Shrinkage of (brain) tissue due to loss of neuronal processes.

attention—The capacity of an individual to screen out certain aspects of the environment and to perceive and process other aspects.

Attention Deficit Disorder (ADD)—ADD is a diagnosis given to children who exhibit the cardinal signs of impulsivity, distractibility, and shortened attention span. These children may also exhibit increased levels of activity in which case the diagnosis of Attention Deficit Hyperactivity Disorder is given.

auditory nerve—Sometimes called the vestibular or acoustic nerve. It is the VIIIth cranial nerve and transmits auditory information and also is involved in the sense of equilibrium. (See also acoustic nerve.)

auditory verbal dysnomia—An aphasic deficit characterized by impairment of the ability to understand the symbolic significance of verbal communication through the auditory avenue (loss of auditory-verbal comprehension).

aura—A sensory or cognitive phenomenon that may precede a seizure.

autonomic nervous system—That part of the nervous system concerned with visceral and involuntary functions.

axon—That portion of a neuron that transmits information from the cell body to the receptors of other neurons.

Babinski response—Extension (instead of flexion) of the toes on stimulation of the sole of the foot, occurring in very young children and in older individuals with lesions of the pyramidal tract.

bacterial infection—Infection by minute, one-celled organisms, which multiply by dividing in one or more directions.

ballismus—An abrupt contraction of the extremities that makes it appear as if the person is flapping or flailing her limbs. It is most commonly seen on one side of the body in which case it is known as hemiballismus. It is sometimes associated with hypotonia and chorea.

basal ganglia—A portion of the brain located within the diencephalon but

Glossary

below the cerebral hemispheres, including the thalamus, caudate nucleus, and lentiform nucleus.
bifurcation—Division into two branches.
Broca's area—A portion of the brain intimately involved in the production of speech.
Capgra's syndrome—A condition wherein the patient is convinced that persons in his close social environment have been replaced with imposters. It is sometimes seen with nondominant hemisphere lesions, posttraumatic encephalopathy, cerebral vascular disease, and other neurological diseases, but usually only in the early stages.
carcinoma—A malignant neoplasm (cancer) that tends to infiltrate surrounding tissue and give rise to metastases
cataplexy—An abrupt decrease in muscle tone. The person feels as if suddenly he has lost control of his limb(s). Can produce falls if the lower limbs are involved.
cerebral anoxia—A condition in which the cells of the brain do not receive sufficient oxygen to perform their normal functions.
cerebral heteropias—Groups of neural cells surrounded by a shell of myelinated fibers. These cells failed to migrate properly and differentiated without being connected to other neural structures.
cerebral palsy—A general term for a large number of congenital neurological disorders. The symptoms include movement disorders, weakness, spasticity, and ataxia. Some degree of mental retardation may also be present. The cause is usually an event during or shortly after the birth process.
cerebrovascular accident—An ischemic disorder that is produced by a disruption of blood flow to the brain due to an occlusion of a portion of the vascular system from a thrombus or embolus or from a hemorrhage.
chorea—a sudden involuntary movement that serves no apparent purpose. These movements are known as choreiform and are brief in duration. They are asymmetric and can often be covered by the afflicted individual unless the examiner is extremely watchful. They are associated with decreased muscle tone.
clonic movements—Spasmodic alteration of contraction and relaxation such as seen in certain forms of epilepsy.
coma—A condition of profound stupor or unconsciousness.
concussion—A form of closed-head injury resulting from a blow to the head or violent shaking of the head.
confabulation—A symptom of Korsakoff's syndrome in which the patient supplies ready answers to questions without regard for the truth. The patient who confabulates appears to "fill in" gaps in memory with plausible facts.
conjugate—Working in unison.

constructional apraxia—See **apraxia**.
constructional dyspraxia—Difficulty in reproducing (drawing) simple geometric design and objects. See **apraxia**.
contralateral—Referring to the opposite side of the body or brain.
contrecoup—Damage in closed head injury that is characterized by destruction of brain tissue opposite the site of impact due to the brain's bouncing off the walls of the cranium.
contusion—A form of closed-head injury that produces mild hemorrahge and associated swelling.
corpus callosum—The brain structure that connects the right and left hemispheres.
cortex—The outer layer of brain tissue comprised of sulci and gyri.
cranial nerves—Twelve pairs of nerves that originate in the brain and carry sensory and motor signals to and from the periphery of the nervous system.
cyst—A sac of fluid usually associated with an infectious disorder.
déjà vu—An experience in which new experiences seem familiar and relived. Feelings of déjà vu are common with complex partial seizures.
delirium—An acute, global impairment of cognitive functioning. It is usually reversible and is due to metabolic disturbance of brain function.
dementia—A condition, usually chronic, of global impairment of cognition which occurs in the absence of clouded consciouness. In some cases, such as in Alzheimer's disease, the condition is progressive.
diplopia—Double vision.
Down syndrome—(Also know as Mongolism or trisomy 21). A condition caused by an abnormality of the 21st chromosome. These children exhibit mental retardation, epicanthal folds around the eyes, and abnormal skeletal growth. Death frequently occurs before the age of 25.
dysarthria—Acquired impairment in motor aspects of speech. Dysarthric speech may sound slurred or compressed. Spastic dysarthria, associated with pseudobulbar palsy, is low in pitch and has a raspy sound with poor articulation. Flaccid dsyarthria, associated with bulbar palsy, has an extremely nasal aspect to its sound. Ataxic dysarthria is associated with cerebellar palsy and has two deficits—articulation and prosody. Hypokinetic dysarthria, found wth parkinsonism, results in low volume speech and less emphasis on accented syllables; there are also articulatory initiation difficulties. Hyperkinetic dysarthria, has prosodic, phonation, and articulatory deficits; the loudness and accents are uncontrolled. There are many disorders that present with combinations of the different types of dysarthria.
dyscalculia—An aphasic symptom characterized by impairment in the ability to appreciate the symbolic significance of numbers and to perform arithmetic calculations.
dysdiadochokinesia—The inability to perform rapid alternating move-

ments. One clinical test for this condition is to ask the patient to hold out both hands and pronate and supinate them as rapidly as possible.

dysfluency—A disturbance of the fluency of speech.

dysgnosia—In contrast to agnosia, dysgnosia represents a partial rather than complete loss of the symbolic significance of information reaching the brain.

dyslexia—See **alexia**.

dysnomia—See **anomia**.

dysphagia—Difficulty in swallowing

dyspnea—Labored breathing.

dyspraxia—See **apraxia**.

dystonia—Involuntary, slow movements that tend to contort a part of the body for a period of time. Dystonic movements tend to involve large portions of the body, and have a sinuous quality that when severe resembles writhing.

echolalia—Repetition of verbal material without apparent knowledge of the meaning.

echopraxia—Mirror copying of the examiner's body movements or positions, especially when under instructions to copy the movements or positions using the same side of the body as does the examiner.

edema—Swelling of tissue following cerebral insult or injury. Cerebral edema results from the accumulation of fluid in intercellular tissue.

embolus—Any foreign object such as an air bubble or blood clot that becomes lodged in a vessel or artery causing an occlusion of blood flow.

encephalitis—Inflammation of the brain.

epilepsy—A condition of abnormal electrical discharges from the brain associated with a temporary alteration in behavior.

eutonia—A general pervasive feeling of well-being.

extrinsic—Outside of the cerebral hemisphere, usually referring to neoplasms or cerebrovascular hemorrhages that are located between the skull and brain.

facial nerve—The VIIth cranial nerve. It is involved in sense of taste and contains a few other somatic sensory afferent fibers. It is also involved in facial expression. Bell's palsy is the result of compression of this nerve.

fissure—Any deep fold in the cerebral cortex. Fissures define the limits of cerbral lobes.

flaccid—Relaxed, flabby, or absent muscle tone.

functional—Having a psychiatric or psychological cause.

gait—The particular manner in which a person moves while walking.

general paresis—Tertiary syphilis, characterized by progressive dementia and generalized paralysis.

glial cells—The connective tissue of the brain (from the Latin word for glue).

glioma—Any neoplasm arising from glial cells.
glossopharyngeal nerve—The IXth cranial nerve consisting largely of sensory afferent fibers. Lesions here might result in the loss of the gag reflex and the carotid sinus reflex, as well as loss of the sense of taste and loss of general sensation in the lower third of the tongue.
gyrus—A convolution on the surface of the brain.
hemianopsia—The loss of vision in one-half of a visual field.
hemiballismus—See **ballismus**.
hemispatial neglect—The failure to detect, report, or orient to one side of the field of experience. Although it is possible with either hemifield, it is much more long lasting when it occurs on the left side. It also know as hemi-inattention or unilateral neglect
hemorrhage—Bleeding.
holoprosencephaly—A condition resulting from the failure of the prosencephalic vesicles in the brain to evaginate. Many of these children are stillborn. If the children survive birth, they are likely to have seizure disorders and spastic weakness of the limbs.
homonymous hemianopsia—The loss of vision in the same half of the visual field in both eyes.
hydrocephalus—A condition marked by accumulation of fluid in the cranium, producing enlarged ventricles and compression of neural tissues.
hyperactivity—Increased levels of behavioral activity. Sometimes associated with ADD.
hypertonia—A state of high muscle tone.
hypoglossal—The XIIth cranial nerve. It has somatic efferent fibers and serves the tongue. Lesions here will result in lower motor neuron loss and contralateral hemiplegia and ipsalateral paralysis of the tongue.
hypothalamus—A structure dorsal to the thalamus that regulates sleeping, sexual activity, eating, emotions, and other behaviors.
hypotonia—A state of low muscle tone. The muscles will feel soft and flabby.
ictal—Related to a seizure (epileptic) episode. For example, cursing is an ictal behavior associated with some forms of temporal lobe epilepsy.
ideational apraxia—See **apraxia**.
ideomotor apraxia—Sometimes called ideokinetic apraxia. See **apraxia**.
idiopathic—A term referring to conditions whose cause is unknown. Epilepsy can be idiopathic or secondary to a known cerebral insult.
infarct—A region of dead brain tissue associated with occlusion of the vasculature.
interictal—Behavior that occurs between seizure episodes in an epileptic individual.
intrinsic—Existing within the brain itself.
ipsilateral—On the same side.

ischemia—Any local and temporary deficiency of blood.

jamais vu—An experience associated with some forms of epilepsy in which familiar surroundings and experiences seem unreal or unusual.

Kayser–Fletcher ring—A brown/green ring around the cornea. This sign is pathognomonic for Wilson's disease.

Korsakoff's syndrome—Deterioration of the brain and cognitive abilities (particularly memory) caused by severe and chronic alcohol abuse and resulting from thiamine deficiency.

Kwashiorkor—A nutritional disorder secondary to a protein-deficient diet. The symptoms include diarrhea, edema, and thin discolored hair and associated cognitive deficits.

learning disability—A decrement in a specific area of academic achievement inconsistent with the intellectual performance of the individual or with other areas of academic achievement.

lesion—Any damage to bodily tissues as a result of disease or injury.

marasmus—A nutritional disorder that is the result of a calorie-deficient diet. The effects include small weight gains during growth, irritability, listlessness, and cognitive deficits.

meninges—Three membranes that protect the brain and provide for venous drainage. The dura mater, pia mater, and arachnoid comprise the cerebral meninges.

meningioma—A neoplasm arising in the meninges.

meningitis—Inflammation of the meninges, especially of the pia mater and the arachnoid.

metastatic neoplasm—A tumor that develops from abnormal cells that have migrated from another part of the body, most commonly from the lungs or breast.

microcephaly—A condition marked by an unusually small brain.

micrographia—Writing with minute letters or on a very small portion of the page.

minimal brain dysfunction—A term sometimes used to refer to a constellation of loosely organized symptoms. It is usually used when the etiology of the symptoms is unknown. It has been used to describe hyperactivity, impulse control, and attention deficits, especially when it is not known for certain if the etiology is in fact organic.

motor impersistence—An inability to continue a motor activity once it is begun despite commands to do so.

multiple sclerosis—A disease resulting from degeneration of myelin, characterized by the development of multiple plaques throughout the brain and spinal cord.

mutism—A condition of not speaking, dumbness. See **akinetic mutism.**

myelopathy—Disintegration of the myelin sheath. Not to be confused with myopathy.

myoclonus—An abrupt contraction of musculature. Myoclonus results in a jerking motion and ordinarily occurs when a person is falling asleep. Myoclonus in the waking stages may be indicative of neuropathology.

myopathy—Degeneration of muscle fiber. Not to be confused with myelopathy.

myotonia—Delayed relaxation of the muscles. Myotonic dystrophy appears in adulthood and is characterized by an inability of the patient to quickly release a grasp or undo any motor contraction. It involves the skeletal muscles.

myxedema—An endocrine disorder in which there is hypofunction of the thyroid resulting in psychomotor slowing, apathy, and drowsiness.

neoplasm—Literally "new growth," the term refers to a tumor.

neuralgia—Acute, paroxysmal pain along the course of a nerve.

neuritis—Inflammation of a nerve.

neurotoxins—Any of a group of chemicals that have negative effects on neural activity. These include some solvents and heavy metals.

nystagmus—A spasmodic movement of the eyes, either rotary or side to side

oculomotor nerve—The IIIrd cranial nerve. It has efferent fibers to the eye muscles. It is responsible for accommodation and pupil dilation among other motor activities. Lesions may result in anisocoria, ptosis, or strabismus.

olfactory nerve—The Ist cranial nerve. It has afferent fibers serving the sense of smell.

optic nerve—The IInd cranial nerve, serving the sense of sight.

pachygyria—A condition marked by decreases in the number of cerebral gyri. In addition, the gyri are broader than usual.

papilledema—Swelling of the optic disk.

paraphasia—A disturbance in the verbal output of a patient. A literal paraphasia involves the substitution of letters in a word, for example, "ridilicous" for "ridiculous." Semantic or verbal paraphasia involves the substitution of one word for another. The two words are usually in the same semantic class, for example, "shirt" for "pants."

parathesia—Abnormalities of sensation especially tactile and somethetic sensation.

Parkinson's disease—A disorder that primarily affects the motor functions of the cerebellum. Parkinson's disease is characterized by tremors and gait disturbance.

pathognomonic signs—Any sign or symptom that is characteristic of a disease or pathological condition and that does not occur in the absence of pathology.

prosopagnosia—An acquired inability to recognize familiar faces usually associated with bilateral posterior lesions (It is different from an inability

Glossary

to recognizes unfamiliar faces which is associated with right posterior lesion.)

pseudodementia—Any form of apparent cognitive impairment that is not global and that mimics dementia. A common form is pseudodementia secondary to depression.

ptosis—Permanent drooping of the upper eyelid.

reduplicative paramnesia—A condition whereby the patient has very strong feelings that the current, novel and unfamiliar environment is actually familiar and personally important. An extremely rare phenomenon.

rigidity—Increased muscle tone that manifests itself as resistance to passive movement.

scanning speech—Slowed speech with pauses between each syllable.

scotoma—A blind or partially blind area in the visual field.

spasm—An involuntary contraction of a muscle group. It can be associated with anxiety or fear as well as with a neurological disorder.

spinal accessory nerve—The XIth cranial nerve. It has efferent fibers for branchiomeric musculature. A lesion here might result in paralysis of the trapezius.

stereognosis—The ability to use tactile cues to recognize objects and shapes.

stereotypy—Repetitive movements that serve no purpose.

strabismus—Lack of muscle coordination such that both eyes cannot be directed to the same object.

stroke—A general term used to describe those disorders of the brain that are characterized by disruption of blood flow.

subdural hematoma—A lesion that results from bleeding into the subdural space.

suppression—Any failure to perceive a stimulus on one side of the body wih bilateral simultaneous stimulation. Suppressions can exist with visual, tactile, or auditory stimulation. Also known as extinction.

synapse—The space between the terminal end of an axon and another cell body. Neurotransmitters are released into the synapse and carry signals from one cell to another.

synkinesia—The involuntary mirroring of movements by muscles not included in the muscles involved in the mirrored, voluntary movements. For example, the mirroring by the left arm of movements made by the right arm.

tentorium—The structure that divides the cerebrum from the cerebellum.

thrombus—Any blood clot that forms in an artery or vessel, creating an occlusion. The thrombus typically forms at the bifurcation of a vessel.

tic—Stereotyped movements which may be simple or complex. They are most commonly found in the muscles of the face and are sensitive to changes in the level of subjective tension.

tinnitus—Ringing in the ears.
tremor—An oscillatory or shaking motion.
trigeminal nerve—The Vth cranial nerve. It has afferent fibers from the face and forehead. It is the conduit for sensation of pain, tactile sensation, and thermal sensation. It also has efferent fibers for the mucous membranes, nose, mouth, teeth, and speech apparatus. It is responsible for the corneal reflex, the tearing reflex, and sneezing.
trochlear nerve—The IVth cranial nerve. It has efferent fibers innervating skeletal muscles. Vertical diplopia is one symptom of a lesion in the trochlear nerve.
unilateral neglect—See **hemispatial neglect**.
vagus—The Xth cranial nerve. It has an inhibitory effect on heart rate. It has several efferent and afferent fibers to the speech apparatus. Lesions here can result in paralysis of the soft palate, pharynx, and larnyx. Possible symptoms include hoarseness, dyspnea, dysphagia, or dysarthria.
ventricles—The spaces within the brain through which cerebrospinal fluid circulates.
vertigo—A sensation of spinning or the perception that external objects are revolving around an individual. Often used somewhat imprecisely to describe a feeling of dizziness.
vorbeireden—A verbal response that is incorrect but that indicates that the patient understood the nature of the question as well as the correct answer.
Wernicke's aphasia—An acquired inablility to communicate verbally due to impairment of receptive abilities. Associated with lesion in the posterior portion of the dominant hemisphere.
Wilson's disease—An autosomal recessive genetic disorder of copper metabolism. Also known as hepatolenticular degeneration.
witzelsucht—Inappropriate jocularity, more commonly found with right hemisphere lesions.

References

Achenbach, T. M. & Edelbrock, C. (1983). *Manual for the Child Behavior Checklist and Revised Child Behavior Profile.* Burlington, VT: University of Vermont.
Alajouanine, T., & Lhermitte, F. (1965). Acquired aphasia in childhood, *Brain, 88,* 653–672.
Alpern, G. D. & Shearer, M. S. (1980). *The Alpern–Boll Developmental Profile II Manual.* Aspen, CO: Psychological Developmental Publications.
Armitage, S. B. (1946). An analysis of certain psychological tests used for the evaluation of brain-injury. *Psychological Monographs, 60.*
Army Individual Test. (1944). Manual of directions and scoring. Washington, D. C.: War Department, Adjutant General's Office.
Atkinson, R. C., & Shiffrin, R. M. (1968). Human memory: A proposed system and its control processes. In K. W. Spence & J. T. Spence (Eds.), *The psychology of learning and motivation: Advances in research and theory* (Vol. 2). New York: Academic Press.
Bannatyne, A. (1974). Diagnosis: a note on recategorization of the WISC scaled scores. *Journal of Learning Disabilities, 7,* 272–274.
Battersby, W. S., Bender, M. B., Pollack, M., & Kahn, R. L. (1956). Unilateral "spatial agnosia" ("inattention") in patients with cortical lesions. *Brain, 35,* 68–93.
Bartel, N. R. (1975). Assessing and remediating problems in language development. In D. Hammill, & N. R. Bartel (Eds.), *Teaching children with learning and behavior problems* (pp. 155–201). Boston: Allyn & Bacon.
Bayley, N. (1969). *Bayley Scales of Infant Development: Birth to two years.* New York: Psychological Corporation.
Beller, H. K. (1970). Parallel and serial stages in matching. *Journal of Experimental Psychology, 84,* 213–219.
Bender, L. (1938). *A visual motor gestalt test and its clinical use* (American Orthopsychiatric Association Research Monographs No. 3).
Benton, A. L. (1967). Problems in test construction in the field of aphasia. *Cortex, 3,* 32–58.
Benton, A. L. (1968). Differential behavioral effects of frontal lobe disease. *Neuropsychologia, 6,* 53–60.
Benton, A. L. (1973). The measurement of aphasic disorders. In A.C. Velasquez (Ed.), *Aspectos patologicos del lengage* (pp. 141–192). Lima: Centro Neuropsicologico.
Benton, A. L (1974). *The Revised Visual Retention Test.* (Fourth Edition). New York: Psychological Corporation.

Benton, A. L. (1980). The neuropsychology of facial recognition. *American Psychologist, 35,* 176–186.
Benton, A. L., Hamsher, K. deS., Varnery, N. R., & Spreen, O. (1983). *Contributions to neuropsychological assessment.* New York: Oxford University Press.
Benton, A. L., Hannay, H. J., & Varney, N. R. (1975). Visual perception of line direction in patients with unilateral brain disease. *Neurology 25,* 907–910.
Benton, A. L., & Van Allen, M. W. (1968). Impairment in facial recognition in patients with cerebral disease. *Cortex , 4,* 344–358.
Berg, E. A. (1948). A simple objective technique for measuring flexibility in thinking. *Journal of General Psychology, 39,* 15–22.
Berg, R., Franzen, M., & Wedding, D. (1987). *Screening for brain impairment: A manual for mental health practice.* New York: Springer.
Billingslea, F. Y. (1963). The Bender-Gestalt: A review and perspective. *Psychological Bulletin, 60,* 233–251.
Binet, A., & Simon, T. (1905). Methodes nouvelles pour le diagnostic du niveau intellectuel des anormaux. *L'Annee Psychologique, 11,* 191–244.
Black, F.W. (1974). WISC Verbal-Performance discrepancies as indicators of neurological dysfunction in pediatric patients. *Journal of Clinical Psychology, 30,* 165–167.
Boder, E. (1973). Developmental dyslexia: A diagnostic approach based on three atypical reading-spelling patterns. *Developmental Medicine and Child Neurology, 15,* 663–687.
Boll, T. J. (1978). Diagnosing brain impairment. In B. B. Wolman (Ed.), *Clinical diagnosis of mental disorders.* New York: Plenum.
Boll, T. J. (1981). The Halstead-Reitan Neuropsychological Battery. In S. B. Filskov, & T. J. Boll (Eds.), *Handbook of clinical neuropsychology* (pp. 577–607). New York: Wiley-Interscience.
Bolter, J. F. (1986). Epilepsy in children: Neuropsychological effects. In J. E. Obrzut & G. W. Hynd (Eds.) *Child neuropsychology: Vol 2 Clinical practice.* Orlando, Florida: Academic Press.
Borod, J. C., Goodglass, H., & Kaplan, E. (1980). Normative data on the Boston Diagnostic Aphasia Examination. *Journal of Clinical Neuropsychology, 2,* 209–216.
Borowski, J. G., Benton, A. L., & Spreen, O. (1967). Word fluency and brain damage. *Neuropsychologia, 5,* 135–140.
Bortner, M., Hertzig, M. E., & Birch, H. G. (1972). Neurological signs and intelligence in brain-damaged children. *Journal of Special Education, 6,* 325–333.
Boyd, T. A., Tramontana, M. G., & Hooper, S. R. (1986). Cross-validation of a psychometric system for screening neuropsychological abnormality in older children. *Archives of Clinical Neuropsychology, 1,* 387-391.
Braine, L. G. (1972). A developmental anlaysis of the effect of stimulus orientation on recognition. *American Journal of Psychology, 85,* 157–187.
Brilliant, P. J., & Gynther, M. D. (1963). Relationships between performance on three tests for organicity and selected patient variables. *Journal of Consulting Psychology, 27,* 474–479.
Buschke, H. (1974a). Two stages of learning by children and adults. *Bulletin of the Psychonomic Society, 2,* 392–394.
Buschke, H. (1974b). Components of verbal learning in children: Analysis by selective reminding. *Journal of Experimental Child Psychology, 18,* 488–498.
Buschke, H., & Fuld, P. A. (1974). Evaluating storage, retention, and retrieval in disordered memory and learning. *Neurology, 24,* 1019–1025.
Byrne, M. C., & Shervanian, C. C. (1977). *Introduction to communicative disorders.* New York: Harper & Row.

Canter, A. (1976). *The Canter Background Interference Procedure for the Bender-Gestalt Test.* Nashville: Counselor Recordings.

Caviness, V. S. (1987) Mental retardation, structural developmental anomalies. In G. Adelman (Ed.) *Encyclopedia of Neuroscience.* Boston: Birkhauser.

Chelune, G. J., & Baer, R. A. (1986). Developmental norms for the Wisconsin card sorting test. *Journal of Clinical and Experimental Neuropsychology, 8,* 219–228.

Clodfelter, C. J., Dickson, A. L., Wilkes, N., & Johnson, R. B. (1987). Alternate forms of selective reminding for children. *The Clinical Neuropsychologist, 1,* 243–249.

Cohen, G. (1972). Hemispheric differences in a letter classification task. *Perception and Psychophysics, 11,* 139–142

Colarusso, R. P., & Hammill, D. D. (1972). *Motor-Free Visual Perception Test.* New York: Psychological Corporation.

Connors, C. (1969) A teacher rating scale for use in drug studies with children. *American Journal of Psychiatry, 126,* 884–888.

Connors, C. K. (1982) Parent and teacher rating forms for the assessment of hyperkinesis in children. In P. A. Keller & L. G. Ritt (Eds.), *Innovations in clinical practice: A source book* (Volume 1, pp. 257–264. Sarasota, Florida, Professional Resource Exchange.

Connors, C. K. & Wells, K. C. (1986). *Hyperkinetic children: A Neuropsychosocial approach.* Beverly Hills, CA: Sage Publications.

Costa, L. D. (1975). The relation of visuospatial dysfunction to digit span performance in patients with cerebral lesions. *Cortex, 11,* 31–36.

Costa, L. D., Vaughan, H. G., Levita, E., Farber, N. (1963). Purdue Pegboard as a predictor of the presence and laterality of cerebral lesions. *Journal of Consulting Psychology, 27,* 133–137.

Das, J. P., Kirby, J. R., & Jarman, R. F. (1975). Simultaneous and successive synthesis: An alternative model for cognitive abilities. *Psychological Bulletin, 82,* 87–103.

Das, J. P., Kirby, J. R., & Jarman, R. F. (1979). *Simultaneous and successive cognitive processes.* New York: Academic Press.

Dean, R. S. (1986). Neuropsychological aspects of psychiatric disorders. In J. E. Obrzut & G. W. Hynd (Eds.) *Child Neuropsychology, Vol. 2 Clinical practice.* Orlando, Florida: Academic Press.

DeMyer, W. (1975). Congenital abnormalities of the central nervous system. In D. B. Tower (Ed.) *The Central nervous system,* Vol. 2, *The Clinical neurosciences.* New York: Raven Press.

Denckla, M. B. (1978). Minimal brain dysfunction. In J. S. Chall & A. F. Mirsky (Eds.), *Education and the Brain.* Chicago: University of Chicago Press.

Dennis, M. (1980). Capacity and strategy for syntactic comprehension after left or right hemidecortication. *Brain and Language, 10,* 287–325.

Dennis, M., & Whitaker, H. A. (1977). Hemispheric equipotentiality and language acquisition. In S. J. Segalowitz and F. A. Gruber (Eds.), *Language Development and Neurological Theory,* New York: Academic Press

DeRenzi, E. (1968). Nonverbal memory and hemispheric side of lesion. *Neuropsychologia, 6,* 181–189.

DeRenzi, E., Pieczuro, A., & Vignolo, L. A. (1968). Ideational apraxia: A quantitative study. *Neuropsychologia, 6,* 41–52.

DeRenzi, E., & Vignolo, L.A. (1962). The Token Test: A sensitive test to detect disturbances in aphasics. *Brain, 85,* 665–678.

DiSimoni, F. (1978). *The Token Test for Children: Manual.* Allen, Texas: DLM-Teaching Resources.

Doll, E. A. (1953). *The measurement of social competence: A manual for the Vineland Social Maturity Scale.* Philadelphia: Educational Test Bureau, Educational Publishers.

Dunn, L. M., & Dunn, L. M. (1981). *Peabody Picture Vocabulary Test–Revised.* Circle Pines, Minnesota: American Guidance Service.

Dunn, L. M., & Markwardt, F. C. Jr. (1970). *Peabody Individual Achievement Test. Manual.* Circle Pines, Minnesota: American Guidance Service.

Dvorine, I. (1953). *Dvorine Pseudo-Isochromatic Plates* (2nd Edition). Baltimore: Waverly Press.

Eisensen, J. (1954). *Examining for aphasia: A manual for the examination of aphasia and related disturbances.* New York: Psychological Corporation.

Eisensen, J. (1973). *Adult Aphasia.* New York: Appleton-Century-Crofts.

Fitzhugh, K. B., Fitzhugh, L. C., & Reitan, R. M. (1962). Wechsler-Bellvue comparison in groups with "chronic" and "current" lateralized and diffuse brain lesions. *Journal of Consulting Psychology, 26,* 306–310.

Fletcher, J. M., Satz, P., & Morris, R. (1982). The Florida Longitudinal Project: A review. In S. A. Mednick & M. S. Harway (Eds.), *Longitudinal projects in the United States* (pp. 313–348). Boston: Nijhoff.

Frankenburg, W. K., & Dodds, J. B. (1967). The Denver Developmental Screening Test. *Journal of Pediatrics, 71,* 181–191.

Frankenburg, W. K., Dodds, J. B., Fandel, A. W., Kazuk, E., & Cohrs, M. (1975). *Denver Developmental Screening Test: Reference manual.* Denver: LADOCA Project and Publishing Foundation.

French, J. L. (1964). *The Pictorial Test of Intelligence.* New York: Houghton Mifflin.

Fuld, P. A. (1975, February). Storage, retention, and retrieval in Korsakoff's syndrome. Presented at International Neuropsychological Society third annual meeting, Tampa, Florida.

Gabel, S., Oster, G. D., & Butnik, S. M. (1986). *Understanding psychological testing in children: A Guide for health professionals.* New York: Plenum.

Gardner, R. A. (1979). *The objective diagnosis of minimal brain dysfunction.* Cresskill, New Jersey: Creative Therapeutics.

Gates, R. D. (1984). Florida Kindergarten Screening Battery (Test Review). *Journal of Clinical Neuropsychology, 6,* 459–465.

Gessell, A. (1949). *Gessell Developmental Schedules.* New York: Psychological Corporation.

Gessell, A., & Amatruda, C. S. (1947). *Developmental diagnosis.* New York: Paul B. Hoeber.

Goehring, M. M., & Majovski, L. V. (1984). Interrater reliability of a clinical neuropsychological screening instrument for adolescents. *International Journal of Clinical Neuropsychology, 6,* 35–41.

Golden, C. J. (1975). A group version of the Stroop Color and Word Test. *Journal of Personality Assessment, 39,* 386–391.

Golden, C. J. (1978). *The Stroop Color and Word Test: A manual for clinical and experimental uses.* Chicago: Stoelting.

Golden, C. J. (1979). *Clinical interpretation of objective psychological tests.* New York: Grune & Stratton.

Golden, C. J. (1981). *Diagnosis and rehabilitation in clinical neuropsychology.* (Second Edition). Springfield, Illinois: Charles C. Thomas.

Golden, C. J. (1987). *Luria-Nebraska Neuropsychological Battery: Children's Revision.* Los Angeles: Western Psychological Services.

Golden, C. J. (1987). *Screening test for the Luria-Nebraska Neuropsychological*

References

Battery: Adult and children's forms. Los Angeles: Western Psychological Services.
Golden, C. J., Hammeke, T. A., & Purisch, A. D. (1985). *The Luria-Nebraska Neuropsychological Battery.* Los Angeles: Western Psychological Services.
Goldman, R., Fristoe, M., & Woodcock, R.W. (1974–1976). *Auditory skills test battery.* Circle Pines, Minnesota: American Guidance Service.
Goldstein, K. (1948). *Aftereffects of brain injuries in war: Their evaluation and treatment.* New York: Grune and Stratton.
Goodglass, H., & Kaplan, E. (1979). Assessment of cognitive deficit in the brain-injured patient. In M. Gazzaniga (Ed.), *Handbook of behavioral neurology* (Vol. 2, *Neuropsychology*). New York: Plenum Press.
Gordon, H. W. (1983). Dyslexia. In R. E. Tarter & G. Goldstein (Eds.), *Neuropsychology of childhood,* New York: Plenum.
Graham, F. K., & Kendall, B. S. (1960). Memory-for-Designs Test: Revised general manual. *Perceptual and Motor Skills, 11*(Supplement 2-VII), 147–188.
Grant, D. A. & Berg, E. A. (1948). A behavioral analysis of degree of reinforcement and ease of shifting to new responses in a Weigl-type card-sorting problem. *Journal of Experimental Psychology, 38,* 401–411.
Gross, A. M. (1985). Children. In M. Hersen & S. M. Turner (eds.) *Diagnostic interviewing.* New York: Plenum Press.
Grundvig, J. L., Needham, W. E., & Ajax, E. T. (1970). Comparisons of different scoring and administration procedures for the Memory-for-Designs Test. *Journal of Clinical psychology, 26,* 353–357.
Guilford, J. P. (1967). *The nature of human intelligence.* New York: McGraw-Hill.
Gutman, E. (1942). Aphasia in childhood. *Brain,* 65, 205–221.
Guy, W. (1976). Physical and neurological examination for soft signs (PANESS). In W. Guy (Ed.) *ECDEU Assessment manual for psychopharmacology* (pp. 384–406.) Rockville, Md: National Institute of Mental Health.
Hain, J. D. (1964). The Bender-Gestalt Test: A scoring method for identifying brain damage. *Journal of Consulting Psychology, 28,* 34–40.
Halstead, W. C. (1947). *Brain and intelligence.* Chicago: University of Chicago Press.
Halstead, W. C., & Wepman, J. H. (1959). The Halstead-Wepman Aphasia Screening Test. *Journal of Speech and Hearing Disorders, 14,* 9–15.
Hannay, H. J., & Levin, H. S. (1985). Selective Reminding Test: An examination of the equivalence of four forms. *Journal of Clinical and Experimental Neuropsychology, 7,* 251–263.
Hartlage, L. C., & Telzrow, C. F. (1983). Neuropsychological Assessment. In K. D. Paget & B. A. Bracker (Eds.), *The psychoeducational assessment of preschool children.* New York: Grune and Stratton.
Hartlage, L. C., & Telzrow, C. F. (1986). *Neuropsychological assessment and intervention with children and adolescents.* Sarasota, Florida: Professional Resource Exchange.
Heaton, R. K. (1981). *Manual for the Wisconsin Card Sorting Test.* Odessa, Florida: Psychological Assessment Resources.
Helton, G. B., Workman, E. A., & Matuszek, P. A. (1982). *Psychoeducational assessment: Integrating concepts and techniques.* New York: Grune & Stratton.
Himelstein, P. (1972). Review of the Slosson Intelligence Test. In O.K. Buros (Ed.), *The seventh mental measurements yearbook* (pp. 424). Highland Park, New Jersey: Gryphon Press.
Hiskey, M. S. (1966). *The Hiskey-Nebraska test of learning aptitude.* Lincoln, Nebraska: Union College Press.

Holroyd, J., & Wright, F. (1965). Neurological implications of WISC Verbal-Performance discrepancies in a psychiatric setting. *Journal of Consulting Psychology, 29,* 206–212.

Horton, K. B. (1974). Infant intervention and language learning. In R. L. Schiefelbusch & L.L. Lloyd (Eds.), *Language perspectives: Acquisition, retardation, and intervention* (pp. 469–491). Baltimore: University Park Press.

Hunt, J. V. (1972). Review of the Slosson Intelligence Test. In O. K. Buros (Ed.), *The seventh mental measurements yearbook* (pp. 424). Highland Park, New Jersey: Gryphon Press.

Hutt, M. (1963). *The Hutt adaptation of the Bender-Gestalt Test.* New York: Grune & Stratton.

Hutt, M. (1969). *The Hutt adaptation of the Bender-Gestalt Test.* (2nd ed.). New York: Grune & Stratton.

Hynd, G. W., Obrzut, J. E., & Obrzut, A. (1981). Are lateral and perceptual asymmetries related to WISC-R and achievement test performance in normal and learning disabled children? *Journal of Consulting and Clinical Psychology, 49,* 977–979.

ILAE (1981). International League Against Epilepsy Commission on classification and terminology: Proposal for revised clinical and electroencephalographic classification of epileptic seizures. *Epilepsia, 22,* 489–501.

Illington, R. S. (1980). *The Development of the infant and young child.* 7th Edition. Edinburgh: Churchill Livingston.

Illington, R. S. (1982). Basic developmental screening 0-4 years, 3rd Edition. Oxford, England: Blackwell Scientific Publication.

Ishihara, S. (1964). *Tests for color blindness* (11th editon). Tokyo: Kanehara Shuppan.

Jarman, R. F., & Nelson, G. (1980). Torque and cognitive ability: Some contributions to Blau's proposals. *Journal of Clinical Psychology, 36,* 458–464.

Jastak, S., & Wilkinson, G. S. (1984). *Wide Range Achievement Test–Revised,* Wilmington, Delaware: Jastak Associates.

Jensen, A. R., & Figueroa, R. A. (1975). Forward and backward digit-span interaction with race and I.Q. *Journal of Educational psychology, 67,* 882–893.

Kaplan, E. F., Goodglass, H., & Weintraub, S. (1978). *The Boston Naming Test.* Boston: E. Kaplan & H. Goodglass.

Karlin, I. W. (1954). Aphasias in children. *American Journal of Disabled Children, 87,* 752–760.

Kaufman, A. S. (1979). *Intelligent testing with the WISC-R.* New York: John Wiley.

Kaufman, A. S., & Kaufman, N. L. (1977). *Clinical evaluation of young children with the McCarthy Scales.* New York: Grune & Statton.

Kaufman, A. S., and Kaufman, N. L. (1983). *Kaufman Assessment Battery for Children,* Circle Pines, Minnesota: American Guidance Service.

Kimura, D. (1963). Right temporal lobe damage. *Archives of Neurology, 8,* 264–270.

Kirk, S. A., McCarthy, J. J., & Kirk, W. D. (1968). *Illinois Test of Psycholinguistic Abilities.* Urbana, Illinois: University of Illinois Press.

Knights, R. M., & Norwood, J. A. (1980). *Revised smoothed normative data on the Neuropsychological Test Battery for Children,* Ottawa, Ontario: Carlton University.

Kohs, S. C. (1927). *Intelligence measurement.* New York : Macmillan.

Koppitz, E. M. (1963). *The Bender Gestalt Test for young children.* New York: Grune & Stratton.

Koppitz, E. M. (1975). *The Bender-Gestalt Test for young children, Volume 2: Research and application, 1963–1973.* New York: Grune & Stratton.

References

Kuhns, J. W. (1979). *Neurological dysfunctions of children.* Monterey, California: Publishers Test Service.
Lambert, N. M., Windmiller, M., Cole, L., & Figueroa, R. A. (1975). Standardization of a public school version and the AAMD Adaptive Behavior Scale. *Mental Retardation, 13,* 3–7.
Lazar, I., & Darlington, R. B. (1978). *Lasting effect after preschool* (DHEW Publication No. OHDS 79-30178). Washington, D.C.: Office of Human Development Services.
Leiter, R. G. (1948). *Leiter International Performance Scale.* Chicago: Stoelting.
Levine, J., & Feirstein, A. (1972). Differences in test performance between brain damaged, schizophrenic, and medical patients. *Journal of Consulting and Clinical Psychology, 39,* 508–520.
Levine, M. D., Busch, B., Aufseeser, C. (1982). The dimension of inattention among children with school problems. *Pediatrics, 59,* 584–587.
Levine, S. C., & Koch-Weser, M. P. (1982). Right hemisphere supcriority in the recognition of famous faces. *Brain and Cognition, 1,* 10–22.
Lezak, M. D. (1982). The problem of assessing executive functions. *International Journal of Psychology, 17,* 281–297.
Lezak, M. D. (1983). *Neuropsychological assessment* (Second Edition). New York: Oxford University Press.
Lowe, J., Krehbiel, R., Sweeney, J., Crumley, K., Peterson, G., Watson, B., & Rhodes, J. (1984). A screening battery for identifying children at risk for neuropsychological deficits: A pilot study. *International Journal of Clinical Neuropsychology, 6,* 42–45.
Ludlow, C. L. (1979). Research directions and needs concerning the neurological bases of language disorders in children. In C. L. Ludlow and M.E. Doran-Quine (Eds.), *The Neurological Bases of Language Disorders in Children: Methods and Directions for Research,* NIH Publication 79–440, Washington, D.C.: U.S. Department of Health, Education, and Welfare.
Luria, A. R. (1966) *Higher cortical functions in man.* New York: Basic Books.
Lutey, C. L. (1967). *Individual intelligence testing: A manual.* Greeley, Colorado: Author.
Majovski, L. V., Tanguay, P., Russell, A., Sigman, M., Crumley, K., & Goldenberg, I. (1979a). Clinical Neuropsychological Screening Instrument for assessment of higher cortical deficits in adolescents. *Clinical Neuropsychology, 1,* 3–8.
Majovski, L. V., Tanguay, P., Russell, A., Sigman, M., Crumley, K., & Goldenberg, I. (1979b). Clinical Neuropsychological Screening Instrument: A clinical research tool for assessment of higher cortical deficits in adolescents. *Clinical Neuropsychology, 1,* 9–19.
Marge, M. (1972). The general problem of language disabilities in children. In J. V. Irwin & M. Marge (Eds.), *Principles of childhood language disabilities,* New York: Appleton-Century-Crofts.
Matarazzo, J. D. (1972). *Wechsler's measurement and appraisal of adult intelligence* (Fifth Edition). Baltimore: Williams & Wilkins.
McCarthy, D. (1972). *McCarthy Scales of Children's Abilities.* New York: Psychological Corporation.
McCarthy, D. (1978). *Manual for the McCarthy Screening Test.* New York: Psychological Corporation.
McFie, J. (1975). *Assessment of organic intellectual impairment.* New York: Academic Press.
McGlone, J. (1985). Can spatial deficits in Turner's syndrome by explained by focal

CNS dysfunction or atypical speech localization? *Journal of Clinical and Experimental* Neuropsychology, 7, 375–394.

Menyuk, P. (1971). *The acquisition and development of language.* Englewood Cliffs, New Jersey: Prentice-Hall.

Milner, B. (1962). Laterality effects in audition. In V.B. Mountcastle (Ed.), *Interhemspheric relations and cerebral dominance* (pp.143–169). Baltimore: Johns Hopkins University Press.

Milner, B. (1967). Brain mechanisms suggested by studies of temporal lobes. In C. H. Millikan & F. L. Darley (Eds.), *Brain mechanisms underlying speech and language* (pp. 25-47). New York: Grune and Stratton.

Moehle, K. A., Berg, R. A., Lancaster, W., & Huck, K. (1985). Statistical test of a short form of the Speech Sounds Perception Test in a child population. *Journal of Clinical Neuropsychology, 6,* 62–64.

Mutti, M., Sterling, H. M., & Spalding, N. V. (1978). *QNST: Quick Neurological Screening Test* (revised edition). Novato, California: Academic Therapy Publications.

Nihira, K., Foster, R., Shellhaas, M., & Leland, H. (1974). *AAMD Adaptive Behavior Scale* (Revised). Washington, D.C.: American Association on Mental Deficiency.

Orton, S. (1937). *Reading, writing, and speech problems in children.* New York: Norton.

Osterrieth, P. A. (1944) La test de copie d'une figure complexe. *Archives de Psychologie, 30,* 206–356.

Palmer, J. O. (1970). *The psychological assessment of children.* New York: John Wiley.

Pascal, G. R., & Suttell, B. J. (1951). *The Bender-Gestalt Test: Quantification and validity for adults.* New York: Grune & Stratton.

Porch, B. E. (1971). Multidimensional scoring in aphasia tests. *Journal of Speech and Hearing Research, 14,* 776–792.

Porteus, S. D. (1959). The *Maze Test and Clinical Psychology.* Palo Alto, California: Pacific Books.

Porteus, S. D. (1965). *Porteus Maze Test: Fifty years' application.* Palo Alto, California: Pacific Books.

Purdue Research Foundation (1948). *Examiner's manual for the Purdue Pegboard.* Chicago: Science Research associates.

Randt, C. T., & Brown, E. R. (1983). *Randt Memory Test.* Bayport, New York: Life Science Associates.

Rapin I. (1982). *Children with brain dysfunction: Neurology, cognition, language, and behavior.* New York: Raven Press.

Rapin, I., Mattis, S., Rowan, A. J., and Golden, G. G. (1977). Verbal auditory agnosia in children. *Developmental Medicine and Child Neurology, 19,* 192–203.

Rapin, I., Tourk, L. M., & Costa, L. D. (1966). Evaluation of the Purdue Pegboard as a screening test for brain damage. *Developmental Medicine and Child Neurology, 8,* 45–54.

Rattan, G. & Dean, R. S. (1985). Quick Neurological Screening Test. In D. J. Keyser & R. C. Sweet (Eds.) *Test Critiques,* Vol. 2, pp. 621–630.

Raven, J. C. (1956). *Guide to using the Coloured Progressive Matrices* (Revised Edition). London: H. K. Lewis.

Raven, J. C. (1960). *Guide to using the Standard Progressive Matrices.* London: H. K. Lewis.

References

Reed, H. B. C. (1976). Pediatric neuropsychology. *Journal of Pediatric Psychology, 1*, 5–7.
Reitan, R. M. (undated). *Instructions and procedures for administering the Neuropsychological Test Battery used at the Neuropsychology Laboratory, Indiana University Medical Center.* Unpublished manuscript.
Reitan, R. M. (1958). Validity of the Trail Making Test as an indicator of organic brain damage. *Perceptual and Motor Skills, 8*, 271–276.
Reitan, R. M. (1955). The distribution according to age of a psychologic measure dependent upon organic brain functions. *Journal of Gerontology, 10*, 330–340.
Reitan, R. M. (1964). Psychological deficits resulting from cerebral lesions in man. In J. M. Warren & K. Akert (Eds.), *The frontal granular cortex and behavior* (pp. 287–306). New York: McGraw-Hill.
Reitan, R. M. (1969). *Manual for administration of neuro–psychological test batteries for adults and children.* Indianapolis, Indiana: Author.
Reitan, R. M. (1974). Methodological problems in clinical neuropsychology. In R. M. Reitan & L. A. Davison (Eds.), *Clinical neuropsychology: Current status and applications.* New York: John Wiley.
Reitan, R. M. (1979). *Manual for administration of neuropsychological test batteries for adults and children.* Tucson, Arizona: Reitan Neuropsychology Laboratories.
Reitan, R. M., & Davison, L.A. (1974). *Clinical Neuropsychology: Current status and applications.* Washington, D.C.: Winston/Wiley.
Reitan, R. M., & Wolfson, D. (1985). *The Halstead-Reitan Neuropsychological Test Battery: Theory and clinical interpretation.* Tucson, Arizona: Neuropsychology Press.
Rey, A. (1941). L'examen psychologique dans les cas d'encephalopathie traumatique. *Archives de Psychologie, 28*, 286–340.
Rey, A. (1964). *L'examen clinique en psychologie.* (English chapter summaries). Paris: Presses Universitaires de France.
Rivara, F. P. & Mueller, B. A. (1986). The epidemiology and prevention of pediatric head injury. *Journal of Head Injury Rehabilitation, 1*(4), 7–15.
Russell, E. W. (1975). A multiple scoring method for the assessment of complex memory functions. *Journal of Consulting and Clinical Psychology, 43*, 800–809.
Russell, E. W., Neuringer, C., & Goldstein, G. (1970). *Assessment of brain damage: A neuropsychological key approach.* New York: John Wiley-Interscience.
Rutter, M. (1982). Syndromes attributed to "minimal brain dysfunction" in childhood. *American Journal of Psychiatry, 139*, 21–33.
Rutter, M., Chadwick, O., & Shaffer, D. (1985). Head injury. In M. Rutter (Ed.) *Developmental neuropsychiatry.* New York: Guilford Press.
Rutter, M., Graham, P., & Yule, W. (1970). *A neuropsychiatric study in childhood.* (C.D.M. Nos. 35/36). London: Heinemann.
Sattler, J. M. (1982). *Assessment of children's intelligence and special abilities* (Second Edition). Boston: Allyn and Bacon.
Sattler, J. M. (in press). *Assessment of children's intelligence and special abilities* (Third Edition). Boston: Allyn and Bacon.
Satz, P., & Bullard-Bates, C. (1981). Acquired aphasia in children. In M. T. Sarno (Ed.), *Acquired Aphasia,* New York: Academic Press.
Satz, P., & Fletcher, J. M. (1982). *Manual for the Florida Kindergarten Screening Battery.* Odessa, Florida: Psychological Assessment Resources.

Satz, P., Taylor, H. G., Friel, J., & Fletcher, J. M. (1978). Some developmental and predictive precursors of reading disabilities: A six-year follow-up. In A. L. Benton & D. Pearl (Eds.), *Dyslexia: An appraisal of current knowledge* (pp. 313–347). New York: Oxford University Press.

Schweinhart, L. J., & Weikart, D. P. (1980). *Young children grow up: The effects of the Perry Preschool Program on youths through age 15*. Ypsilanti, Michigan: Monographs of the High/Scope Education Research Foundation.

Seashore, C. E., Lewis, D., & Saetveit, D. L. (1960). *Seashore measures of musical talents* (revised editon). New York: Psychological Corporation.

Sergent, J., & Bindra, D. (1981). Differential hemispheric processing of faces: Methodological considerations and reinterpretation. *Psychological Review, 89*, 541–554.

Shaffer, D., O'Connor, P. A., Shafer, S. Q., & Prupis, S. (1983). Neurological "soft signs:" Their origins and significance for behavior. In M. Rutter (Ed.), *Developmental neuropsychiatry*, New York: Guiford Press.

Simenson, R. J., & Sutherland, J. (1974). Psychological assessment of brain damage: The Wechsler scales. *Academic Therapy, 10*, 69–81.

Simmons, J. E. (1987). *Psychiatric examination of children*, 4th Edition. Philadelphia: Lea & Febiger.

Slosson, R. L. (1963). *Slosson Intelligence Test (SIT) for Children*. New York: Slosson Educational Publications.

Smith, A. (1960). Changes in Porteus Maze scores of brain-operated schizophrenics after an eight year interval. *Journal of Mental Science, 106*, 967–978.

Smith, A., & Kinder, E. (1959). Changes in psychological test performances of brain-operated subjects after eight years. *Science, 129*, 149–150.

Sparrow, S. S., Balla, D. A., & Cicchetti, D. V. (1984). *Vineland Adaptive Behavior Scales*. Circle Pines, Minnesota: American Guidance Service.

Spreen, O., & Benton, A. L. (1969). *Neurosensory Center Comprehensive Examination for Aphasia*. Victoria, B. C.: Neuropsychology Laboratory. Department of Psychology, University of Victoria.

Spreen, O., Tupper, D., Risser, A., Tuokko, H., & Edgell, D. (1984). *Human Developmental Neuropsychology*, New York: Oxford University Press.

Springer, S. P., & Deutsch, G. (1981). *Left brain, right brain*. San Francisco: W. H. Freeman.

Stamm, J. S. & Kreder, S. V. (1979). Minimal brain dysfunction: Psychological and neurophysiological disorders in hyperkinetic children. In M. S. Gazzaniga, *Neuropsychology*. Vol. 2 of *Handbook of Behavioral Neurology* (F.A. King, Ed.). New York: Plenum.

Sterling, H. M., & Sterling, P. J. (1977). Experiences with the QNST (Quick Neurological Screening Test). *Academic Therapy, 12*, 339–342.

Sterne, D. M. (1966). The Knox cubes as a measure of memory and intelligence with adult males. *Journal of Clinical Psychology, 22*, 191–193.

Stone, M. H. & Wright, B. D. (1980). *Knox's Cube test instruction manual*. Chicago: Stoelting.

Street, R. F. (1931). A Gestalt Completion test. *Contributions to education*, No. 481. New York: Bureau of Publications, Teachers College, Columbia University.

Stroop, J. R. (1935). The basis of Ligon's theory. *American Journal of Psychology, 47*, 499–504.

Talley, J. L. (1987). Memory in learning disabled children: Digit Span and the Rey Auditory Verbal Learning Test. *Archives of Clinical Neuropsychology, 1*, 315–322.

References

Teeter, P. A. (1986). Standard neuropsychological batteries for children. In J. E. Obrzut, & G. W. Hynd (Eds.), *Child Neuropsychology, Volume 2: Clinical Practice* (pp. 187–228). New York: Academic Press.

Terman, L. M., & Merrill, M. A. (1973). *Stanford-Binet Intelligence Scale. Manual for the third revision.* Boston: Houghton Mifflin.

Teuber, H. L., & Rudel, R.G. (1962). Behavior after cerebral lesions in children and adults. *Developmental Medicine and Child Neurology, 4,* 3–20.

Tharp, B. R. (1987). An overview of pediatric seizure disorders and epileptic syndromes. *Epilepsia, 28,* (Suppl. 1) s36–245.

Thorndike, R. L., Hagen, E. P., & Sattler, J. M. (1986). *The Stanford-Binet Intelligence Scale: Fourth Edition, Guide for administering and scoring.* Chicago: Riverside Publishing Company.

Tolor, A., & Schulberg, H. (1963). *An evaluation of the Bender-Gestalt.* Springfield, Illinois: Charles C. Thomas.

Touwen, B. C. L. (1987). The meaning and value of soft signs in neurology. In D. E. Tupper (Ed.) *Soft neurological signs.* Orlando, Fla: Grune & Stratton.

Tramontana, M. G., & Boyd, T. A. (1986). Psychometric screening of neuropsychological abnormality in older children. *International Journal of Clinical Neuropsychology, 8,* 53-59.

Tramontana, M. G., Klee, S. H., & Boyd, T. A. (1984). WISC-R interrelationships with the Halstead-Reitan and Children's Luria Neuropsychological Batteries. *International Journal of Clinical Neuropsychology, 6,* 1–8.

Tupper, D. E. (1986). Neuropsychological screening and soft signs. In J. E. Obrzut & G. W. Hynd (Eds.), *Child Neuropsychology: Volume 2, Clinical Practice.* New York: Academic Press.

Tzavaras, A., Hecaen, H., & LeBras, H. (1970). Le probleme de la specificite du deficit de la reconnaissance du visage humain lors des lesions hemispheriques unilaterales. *Neuropsychologia, 8,* 403–416.

Waber, D. P., & Holmes, J. M. (1985). Assessing children's copy productions of the Rey-Osterrieth Complex Figure. *Journal of Clinical and Experimental Neuropsychology, 7,* 264–280.

Waber, D. P., & Holmes, J. M. (1986). Assessing children's memory productions of the Rey-Osterrieth Complex Figure. *Journal of Clinical and Experimental Neuropsychology, 8,* 563–580.

Warrington, E. K., & James, M. (1967). Disorders of visual perception in patients with localized cerebral lesions. *Neuropsychologia, 5,* 253–266.

Wasserstein, J., Weiss, E., Rosen, J., Gerstman, L., & Costa, L. (January 1980). Reexamination of Gestalt completions tests: Implications for right hemisphere assessment. Presented at the International Neuropsychological Society annual meeting, San Francisco, California.

Wechsler, D. (1939). *Manual for the Wechsler-Bellvue Intelligence Scale.* New York: Psychological Corporation.

Wechsler, D, & Stone, C. P. (1945). *Manual for the Wechsler-Memory Scale.* New York: Psychological Corporation.

Wechsler, D., & Stone, C. P. (1987). *Manual for the Wechsler-Memory Scale-Revised.* New York: Psychological Corporation.

Wechsler, D. (1949). *Manual for the Wechsler Intelligence Scale.* New York: Psychological Corporation.

Wechsler, D. (1955). *Manual for the Wechsler Adult Intelligence Scale.* New York: Psychological Corporation.

Wechsler, D. (1967). *Manual for the Wechsler Preschool and Primary Scale of Intelligence.* New York: Psychological Corporation.

Wechsler, D. (1974). *Manual for the Wechsler Intillegence Scale for Children—Revised.* New York: Psychological Corporation.

Wechsler, D. (1981). *Manual for the Wechsler Adult Intelligence - Revised.* New York: Psychological Corporation.

Weinberg J., Diller, L., Gerstman, L., & Schulman, P. (1972). Digit span in right and left hemiplegics. *Journal of Clinical Psychology, 28,* 361.

Wells, F. L., & Ruesch, J. (1969). *Mental examiner's handbook* (Revised Edition), New York: Psychological Corporation.

Werner, E. E. (1972). Review of the Denver Developmental Screening Test. In O. K. Buros (Ed.), *The seventh mental measurements yearbook* (pp.734–736). Highland Park, New Jersey: Gryphon Press.

Wilkening, G. N., & Golden, C. J. (1982). Pediatric Neuropsychology: Status, theory, and research. In P. Karyoly, & D. O'Grady (Eds.), *Child health psychology: Concepts and issues* (pp.132–167). New York: Pergamon Press.

Williams, D. T., Pleak, R., & Hanesian, H. (1987). Neuropsychiatric disorders of childhood and adolescence. In R.E. Hales & S. C Yudofsky (Eds.) *Textbook of Neuropsychiatry.* Washington, D. C.: American Psychiatric Press, Inc.

Wilson, B. C. (1986). An approach to the neuropsychological assessment of the preschool child with developmental deficits. In S. B. Filskov, & T. J. Boll (Eds.), *Handbook of clinical neuropsychology* Volume 2 (pp. 121–171).

Wilson, B. C., Iacoviello, J. M., Wilson, J. J., & Risucci, D. (1982). Purdue Pegboard performance in normal preschool children. *Journal of Clinical Neuropsychology, 4,* 19–26.

Wirt, R. D., Lachar, D., Klinedinst, J. K. & Seat, P. D. (1984). *Multidimensional description of child personality: A Manual for the Personality Inventory for Children* (Revised by D. Lachar.) Los Angeles: Western Psychological Services.

Wolf, B. A., & Tramontana, M. G. (1982). Aphasia Screening Test interrelationships with complete Halstead-Reitan test results for older children. *Clinical Neuropsychology, 4,* 179–186.

Wysocki, J. J., & Sweet, J. J. (1985). Identification of brain-damaged, schizophrenic, and normal medical patients using a brief neuropsychological screening battery. *International Journal of Clinical Neuropsychology, 7,* 40–44.

Index

Academic achievement, 8
  equivalent scores, 9
  grade equivalencies, 9
  standardized tests, 56
  testing, 9
  T-scores, 9
  Z-scores, 9
Academic skills assessment, 150
  See also History, academic;
  Specific tests
Academic Skills Disorders, 37
Achenbach, T. M., 60
Achenbach Child Behavior Checklist, 60
Adaptive behavior screening, *see* Social behavior screening
Advanced Progressive Matrices, 116
Affective disorders, 34–35, 67
Aggression, 34
Agnosia,
  spatial, 108
  visual, 87
Ajax, E. T., 165
Alajouanine, T., 137
Alcohol, maternal use of, 19–20
Alpern, G. D., 64
Alpern-Boll developmental schedule, 64
Amatruda, C. S., 191
American Association on Mental Deficiency (AAMD), 13
  Adaptive Behavior Scale (ABS), 197–198
  scoring, 197
American Association on Mental Deficiency (AAMD) Adaptive Behavior Scale (ABS) Public School Version, 197, 198
Anxiety disorders, 35
Aphasia, 110
  childhood, 136–138
  childhood vs. adult aphasia, 137
  tests, *See also specific tests* 138–147
Aphasia Screening Test (AST), 120, 138
  Spatial Relations, 182, 183
  stimulus figures, 139
  test items (ages 5–8), 142–143
  test items (ages 9–14), 140–141
Apnea, 42
Armitage, S. B., 181
Army Individual Test, 108
Atkinson, R. C., 92
Attention, 73–74, 159
  and mental status exam description, 74
  vigilance, 74
Attention Deficit Disorder (ADD), 36–37, 42–43
  and dysfunction theories, 36
  features, 36
  symptoms, 43
  treatment, 36
Audiology, 133
Auditory disorders, 21
Auditory Functions assessment, *See also specific tests* 118–121
Auditory perception testing, 147

Babbling, 134
Baer, R. A., 127
Balla, D. A., 198

Bannatyne, A., 84, 85, 86
Bartel, N. R., 134
Battersby, W. S., 107
Bayley, N., 193
Bayley Scales of Infant Development, 191, 193–194
  Infant Behavior Record, 193, 194
  Mental Development Index, 194
  Mental Scale, 193–194
  Motor Scale, 193, 194
  problems, 194
  Psychomotor Development Index, 194
Beery Developmental Test of Visual-Motor Integration (DVMI), 184
Behavioral pediatrician,
  definition, 6
  evaluation, 6
Beller, H. K., 92
Bender, L., 110, 111, 112, 114
Bender, M. B., 107
Bender Visual-Motor Gestalt Test, 109–115, 164, 180
  disadvantages, 112, 115
  Koppitz's scoring, 112, 113, 114
  sample, 111
  scoring systems, 112–115
  success statistics, 115
Benton, A. L., 93, 108, 117, 137, 143, 148, 149, 166
Benton Visual Retention Test (BVRT), 78, 166–167
  scoring, 166
Berg, E. A., 126
Berg, R. A., 73, 110, 121, 147
Billingslea, F. Y., 115
Bindra, D., 93, 97
Binet, A., 94
Birch, H. G., 81
Black, F. W., 81
Boder, E., 150, 151

Boder's Diagnostic Screening Procedure, 150
  scoring, 150
Boll, T. J., 126, 131
Borod, J. C., 148
Borowski, J. G., 149
Bortner, M., 81
Boston Diagnostic Aphasia Examination, Cookie Theft Picture, 149
Boston Naming Test, 148
Boyd, T. A., 188, 189
Braine, L. G., 93
Brillant, P. J., 115
Brown, E. R., 159
Bullard-Bates, C., 137
Buschke, H., 161, 162
Butnik, S. M., 84, 110, 191, 193, 194, 195, 198, 199
Byrne, M. C., 134

Canter, A., 115
Category Test, 125–126, 180
Caviness, V. S., 27
Central nervous system disorder, mental status exam, 72
Cerebral palsy, 30
  causes, 30
  definition, 6
Cerebral vascular accident, mental status, 72
Chadwick, O., 31
Chehine, G. J., 127
Child abuse, 58
Child neuropsychologist, 3, 7–8, 10, 15, 22
  evaluation, 8
  training, 7, 178
Children's Neuropsychological Screening Test (CNST), 188
Cicchetti, D. V., 198
Child psychiatrist, 3, 7, 28
  evaluation, 7

Index

training, 7
Child psychologist, 16
Choreiform movement, 47
Clinical Neuropsychological Evaluation (CNE), 187–188
  scoring, 187
Clodfelter, C. J., 161
Close, J., 49
Cognitive abilities, general screening devices, 191–196
Cognitive function assessment, 124–129
Cohen, G., 92
Cohrs, M., 191
Colarusso, R. P., 106
Cole, L., 197
Color blindness, 105
Color Form Test, 181
Color Perception, 105–106
Color Sorting Test, 106
Coloured Progressive Matrices, 115–116
Conduct disorders, 34
Connors, C. K., 36
Constructional abilities, 78–79
Controlled Word Association Test, 149
Cortico-behavioral function, 9
Costa, L. D., 94, 131, 156
Crumley, K., 187, 188

Darlington, R. B., 190
Das, J. D., 91, 92, 94
Davison, L. A., 126, 129, 131, 138, 157
Dean, R. S., 34
Dementia, 14, 27
Denail, 17, 20
Dennis, M., 137
Denver Development Screening Test (DDST), 191
DeRenzi, E., 141, 147, 164, 173
Deutsch, G., 96, 98

Developmental Arithmetic Disorder, 38
Developmental Coordination Disorder, 36
Developmental delay, definition, 12
Developmental disorders, 12–22
  Developmental Articulation Disorder, 22
  Developmental Expressive Language Disorder, 22
  Developmental Expressive Writing Disorder, 22, 38
  Developmental Reading Disorder, 22, 38
Developmental Screening Inventory (DSI), 191–192
Developmental soft signs,
  associated movements, 44
  detection of, 45
  motor awkwardness, 44, 45
  motor impersistance, 45. *See also* Test of Motor Impersistance
  tactile extinction, 46
Dickson, A. L., 161
Diller, L., 94
DiSimoni, F., 146
Dodds, J. B., 191
Down's Syndrome, 14–15, 17
  cause, 17
  profile, 17
  treatment, 17
DSM-III R, 13, 22, 36, 37, 42, 68
Dunn, L. M., 107, 146, 151
Dvorine, I., 106
Dvorine Screening Test, 106
Dysgraphias, 108
Dyslexia, 38, 108, 125
  developmental, 150
Dyslexics,
  dyseidetic, 151
  dysphonetic, 151

Dyslexics (*continued*)
  mixed dysphonetic-dyseidetic (alexia), 151
Dysphasia, 136. *See also* Aphasia

Eating disorders, 35
Echolalia, 35, 134
Edelbrock, C., 60
Edgell, D., 135, 136
Eisensen, J., 138, 147
Emotional/behavioral patterns, mental status exam, 72
Emotional disorders, 21
Environmental toxins, lead paint chips, 18, 155
Equation for screening neuropsychological abnormality, 188
Epilepsy, 6, 24, 26
  localization-related, 24, 25
  seizures, 61
Evaluative instruments,
  interview, xii, 53–60
  medical history, xi, xii, 67–68
  mental status exam, xi, xii, 70–79
Expressive disorders, screening, 149

Face recognition, 107–108
Fandel, A. W., 191
Farber, N. 131
Feirstein, A., 115
Figueroa, R. A., 94, 197
Finger Oscillation Test, 129, 131
Finger Tapping Test, 129, 130, 181
Fingertip Symbol Writing Recognition test, 124
Fitzhugh, K. B., 190
Fitzhugh, L. C., 190
Fletcher, J. M., 184
Florida Kindergarten Screening Battery (FKSB), 184–185, 186
  Alphabet Recitation Test, 184
  Finger Localization Test, 184
  Recognition-Discrimination measure, 184
Foster, R., 197
Frankenburg, W. K., 191
Franzen, M., 73, 110, 121
French, J. L., 117
Friel, J., 184
Fristoe, M., 121
Fuld, P. A., 162

Gabel, S., 84, 110, 153, 191, 193, 195, 198, 199
Gates, R. D., 185
Genetic disorders, 15–17. *See also* Down's syndrome; Phenylketonuria (PKU); Turner's syndrome
Gerstman, L., 94
Gesell, A., 191, 192
Goehring, M. M., 187
Golden, C. J., 87, 88, 99, 104, 105, 108, 120, 124, 182, 186, 187
Golden, G. G., 137
Goldenberg, I., 187, 188
Goldman, R., 121
Goldman-Fristoe-Woodcock (GFW) Auditory Diagnostic Battery, 121
  Auditory Selective Attention Test, 121
Goldstein, K., 95
Goodglass, H., 148, 149
Gordon, H. W., 96
Graham, F. K., 164
Grant, D. A., 126
Greek Cross, *see* Aphasia Screening Test, Spatial Relations
Grip Strength test, 131
Gross, A. M., 55
Grundvig, J. L., 165

Index

Guilford, J. P., 85, 86
Gutman, E., 137
Gynther, M. D., 115

Hagen, E. P., 157, 195
Hain, J. D., 112
Halstead, W. C., 120, 135, 129, 138, 171, 181, 182
Halstead-Reitan Neuropsychological Battery, 138
Halstead-Reitan Neuropsychological Test Battery for Adults, 109–110
Halstead-Reitan Neuropsychological Test Battery for Children, 177
Halstead and Wepman Aphasia Screening Test, *see* Aphasia Screening Test (AST)
Hammeke, T. A., 182
Hammill, D. D., 106
Hand dynamometer, 131
Hanesian, H., 28
Hannay, H. J., 161
Hard signs, 39
Hartlage, L. C., 97, 193, 197
Head injury, 30–32, 34, 59, 61. *See also* Hematoma
  mental health exam, 72
  prevention, 32
  statistics, 30
Hearing disorders, 12
Heaton, R. K., 127
Hecaen, H., 108
Helton, G. B., 195
Hematoma, 30
Hertzig, M. E., 81
Himelstein, P., 193
Hiskey, M. S., 163
Hiskey-Nebraska Test of Learning Aptitude, Visual Attention Span subtest, 163

History,
  academic, 65–66. *See also* Interview, with school personnel
  developmental, 63–65
  family, 62
  genetic, 60
  medical, 67–68
  occupational, 66–67
  prenatal, 62–63
  sexual, 67
Holmes, J. M., 170, 171
Holroyd, J., 81
Hooper, S. R., 189
Horton, K. B., 190
Huck, K., 147
Hunt, J. V., 192, 193
Hutt, M., 110, 112
Hydrocephalus, 26–27
  cause, 26
  communicating, 26
  features, 27
  noncommunicating, 26
  treatment, 27
Hynd, G. W., 81
Hyperactivity, 42
Hypersexuality, 67
Hypokinesis, 47
Hypoxia, 42

Iacoviello, J. M., 131
Ideational dyspraxia, testing, 147
Illinois Test of Psycholinguistic Abilities, 157
  Visual Association subtest, 118
  Visual Sequential Memory subtest, 163
Incoordination, significant, 47
Infantile autism, 35–36
  diagnosis, 35
Intelligence tests, 13, 64. *See also specific types of tests*

International League Against
  Epilepsy, 24
Interview, 53–60
  with child, 53–58
  clinician-child relationship, 54
  language, 54, 55–56
  questions, 57
  parent-child relationship, 55
  with parents, 58–59
  sample form, 200–204
  with school personnel, 59–60,
    65, 159. *See also* History,
    academic setting, 57
  and social relationships, 56
  structure, 54, 68
Ishihara, S., 54, 68, 106
Ishihara Screening Test, 106

James, M., 107
Jarman, R. F., 92, 94
Jastak, S., 98, 152
Jensen, A. R., 94
Johnson, R. B., 161
Judgment of Line Orientation, 117

Kaplan, E. F., 148, 149
Karlin, I. W., 137
Kaufman, A. S., 81, 82, 84, 85, 86,
  90, 91, 92, 93, 94, 96, 97,
  108, 157
Kaufman, N. L., 90, 91, 92, 93, 94,
  96, 97, 108, 157
Kaufman Assessment Battery for
  Children, xii, 90–99, 103, 157
  Achievement scale, 92, 96, 97,
    98
  Mental Processing, 92
  Nonverbal Scale, 92
  purpose, 90
  scoring, 92
  Sequential Processing, 90, 91,
    93, 94, 95

Simultaneous Processing, 90, 91,
  92, 93, 94, 95, 96
Kaufman Assessment Battery for
  Children subtests, 92
  Arithmetic, 97–98
  Expressive vocabulary, 96–97
  Faces and Places, 97
  Facial recognition, 93, 108
  Gestalt closure, 94
  Hand movements, 87
  Magic Window, 92, 93
  Matrix analogies, 95
  Number recall, 94
  Photo series, 96
  Reading/Decoding, 98
  Reading/Understanding, 98–99
  Riddles, 98
  Spatial memory, 96
  Triangles, 94–95
  Word Order, 95
Kazuk, E., 191
Kendall, B. S., 164
Kimura, D., 163
Kinder, E., 129
Kirby, J. R., 92, 94
Kirk, S. A., 118, 157, 163
Kirk, W. D., 118, 157, 163
Klee, S. H., 188
Klinedinst, J. K., 60
Knights, R. M., 172
Knox Cube Test, 165–166
  scoring, 165
Koch-Weser, M. P., 97
Kohs, S. C., 95
Kohs' Block Design Test, 95
Koppitz, E. M., 112, 113, 114
Kreder, S. V., 36
Krehbiel, R., 188
Kuhns, J. W., 48

Lachar, D., 60
Lambert, N. M., 197
Lancaster, W., 147

Language development, normal, 134–135
Language disorders, 21, 107, 133, 135–136
  DSM-III R, 22
  expressive speech "deficits," 21
  receptive "deficits," 31
Language skills, 74–77
  auditory discrimination, 75
  comprehension, 75
  elements, 76
  expressive, 75
  mental status exam, 75–76
  receptive, 75
Lazar, I., 190
Learning disabilities, definition, 43
Learning disorders, 37–38
LeBras, H., 108
Leiter, R. G., 196
Leiter International Performance Scale, 196
Leland, H., 197
Levin, H. S., 161
Levine, J., 115
Levine, S. C., 97
Levita, E., 131
Lewis, D., 120
Lezak, M. D., 95, 127, 128, 148, 149, 152, 153, 154, 156, 167, 169
Lhermitte, F., 137
Lowe, J., 188
Ludlow, C. L., 137
Luria, A. R., 91, 92, 93, 95, 103
Luria-Nebraska, Battery—Children's Revision, Rhythm Scale, 120
Luria-Nebraska Neuropsychological Battery, 177, 183
  Pathognomonic Scale, 176, 177
  statistics, 177
Luria-Nebraska Neuropsychological Battery Screening Test, 186–187
  scoring, 186–187
Luria's theory of neuropsychological development, 104–105
Lutey, C. L., 159

Majovski, L. V., 187, 188
Marge, M., 135
Markwardt, F. C., Jr., 151
Matarazzo, J. D., 82
Mattis, S., 137
Matuzek, P. A., 195
Maze tests, 123–125, 127–129
  Porteus Maze, 127, 128
  Porteus Maze Extension, 128
  Porteus Maze Supplement, 128
  Vineland Revision, 127
McCarthy, D., 117, 160, 185
McCarthy, J. J., 118, 157, 163
McCarthy Scales of Children's Abilities, 185
  Conceptual Grouping, 186
  Draw-a-Design, 185–186
  Leg Coordination, 186
  Numerical Memory, 186
  Puzzle Solving subtest, 117
  Right-Left Orientation, 185
  scoring, 186
  Verbal Memory, 185
  Verbal Memory 1, 160
  Verbal Memory 2, 160
McCarthy Screening Test, 185–186
McFie, 117
Memory, J., 77–78
  associative, 77
  delayed, 77
  long-term, 77
  recall, 78
  recognition, 78
  short-term, 77
  verbal, 78
  visual, 77, 78

Memory for Designs Test, 164–165
  scoring, 164–165
Mental retardation, 12, 29
  causes, 14, 15
  effect of labelling, 14
  mental status exam, 72
  profile, 13
  requirements for diagnosis, 13
Mental status exam, 70–79, 154
  assessment, 71
  attention, 73–74
  central nervous system disorder, 72
  cerebral vascular accident, 72
  constructional abilities, 78–79
  description, 71
  emotional/behavioral patterns, 72
  head injury, 72
  language, 74–77
  memory, 77–78
  and mental retardation, 72
  and psychiatric symptoms, 72
  purpose, 70
  and sensory function, 72
  standard procedures, 70
  success outcome, 70, 73
Menyuk, P., 134
Merrill, M. A., 148, 149
Milner, B., 118, 119, 148
Minimal brain dysfunction (MBD), 40
Moehle, K. A., 149
Morris, R., 184
Motor disorders, 29
  symptoms, 29
Motor-Free Visual Perception Test (MVPT), 106
Motor Function assessment, 129–132
Muscular dystrophy, 28–29
  and mental retardation, 29
  types of, 28, 29

National Institute of Mental Health, 49
Needham, W. E., 165
Nelson, G., 92
Neurological disorders, *see specific types of disorders*
Neurological dysfunction, 81, 82
Neurological Dysfunction of Children (NDOC), 48
  scoring system, 48
  strengths, 48
  validity studies, 49
Neurological hard signs, *see* Hard signs
Neurological soft signs, *see* Soft signs
Neuropsychology, 133
Neuropsychological screening battery, purpose, 180
Neurotoxins, 17–18, 35
Nihira, K., 197
Norwood, J. A., 172
Nutrition deficiency, 18–20
  vitamin A, 19
  kwashiorkor, 19
  marasmus, 19
  thiamine (vitamin B_1), 18–19
Nystagmus, 47

Obrzut, A., 81
Obrzut, J. E., 81
Oromotor apraxia, 47
Orton, S., 38
Oster, G. D., 84, 110, 191, 193, 195, 198, 199
Osterrieth, P. A., 167, 168, 169, 170

Index

Paired Associates Tasks, 159
  Randt Memory Test, 159
  Wechsler Memory Scale, 159
  Wechsler Memory Scale-Revised, 159
Palmer, J. O., 114
Pascal, G. R., 112
Peabody Individual Achievement Test (PIAT), 151
Peabody Individual Achievement Test (PIAT) subtest,
  General Information, 152
  Mathematics, 152
  Reading Comprehension, 152
  Reading Recognition, 152
  Spelling, 152
Peabody Picture Vocabulary Test-Revised (PPVT-R), 107, 146–147, 151, 184
  scoring, 146
Pediatrician, 3, 5
  definition, 5
  training, 5
Pediatric neurologist, 3, 6, 15, 28, 45
  definition, 6
  evaluation, 6
Perceptual functioning, 107
Personality Inventory for Child, 60
Peterson, G., 188
Phenylketonuria (PKU), 15–16
  features, 15
  phenylalanine, 15
  profile, 16
  treatment, 16
Physical and Neurological Examination for Soft Signs (PANESS), 49
  description, 49
  reliability, 49
  scoring, 49
Pica, 18, 35

Pictorial Test of Intelligence, Similarities subtest, 117–118
Picture recognition, 107
Pieczuro, A., 147
Pleak, R., 28
Porch, B. E., 147
Porteus, S. D., 127, 128
Progressive Figures Test, 181
Psychoeducational evaluation, 10
Psychiatric disorders, symptoms, 33
Psychiatric symptoms, and mental status exam, 72
Psychological Corporation, 159
Psychological intervention, need for, 13
Purdue Pegboard, 131–132
Purdue Research Foundation, 131
Purisch, A. D., 182

Questionnaire, 60
  Achenbach Child Behavior Checklist, 60, 65
  Personality Inventory for Child, 60, 65
Quick Learning Disability Screening Test, 50
Quick Neurological Screening Test (QNST), 50

Random Letters Procedure, 74
Randt, C. T., 159
Rapin, I., 131, 137
Raven, J. C., 95, 114
Raven's Progressive Matrices, 95, 114, 115
Reading disorders, 150
Recall, 159
Recurring Figures Test, 163–164
Reed, H. B. C., 82

Reitan, R. M., 95, 108, 109, 122, 126, 129, 131, 138, 157, 173, 181, 182, 190
Reitan-Indiana Aphasia Screening Test, 188, 189
Reitan-Indiana Neuropsychological Test Battery for Young Children, 177
  Color Form Test, 181, 182
  Progressive Figures Tests, 181, 182
Reitan-Klove Sensory Perceptual Examination, 121–122
  sample form, 122
  scoring, 122
Remedial educational program, 10
Restricted reminding, 162
Restricted reminding tests, 162
Rey, A., 157, 167
Rey Auditory-Verbal Learning Test, xii, 157–158
  scoring, 158
  Test Words, 157
Rey-Osterrieth Complex Figure Test, 167–171
  scoring, 169, 170
Rhodes, J., 188
Risser, A., 135, 136
Risucci, D., 131
Rosen, J., 94
Rowan, A. J., 137
Rudel, R. G., 104
Ruesch, J., 149
Russell, A., 187, 188
Rutter, M., 31

Saetveit, D. L., 120
Sattler, J. M., 81, 83, 84, 87, 88, 157, 193, 195, 196, 198
Satz, P., 137, 184
Schizophrenia, 34
School psychologist, 5, 8, 10
  evaluation, 8
  training, 8
Schulberg, H., 115
Schulman, P., 94
Schweinhart, L. J., 190
Screening Batteries vs. Single Tests vs. Comprehensive Test Batteries, 177–181
Seashore, C. E., 120
Seashore Rhythm Test, 120
Seat, P. D., 60
Seizure disorders, 23–26
  causes, 24
  classification systems, 24, 25
  idiopathic, 24
Seizures,
  absence seizure, 25
  complex-partial symptoms, 25
  idiopathic, 25
  motor, 25
  myoclonic, 25
  psychological causes, 26
  simple-partial, 25
Selective Reminding Test, 160–162
  sample form, 161
Sensory disorders, 20–21
Sensory function, and mental status exam, 72
Sequin-Goddard Formboard, 171
Sergent, J., 93, 97
Sexual abuse, 59
Shaffer, D., 31
Shearer, M. S., 64
Shellhaas, M., 197
Shervanian, C. C., 134
Shiffrin, R. M., 92
Sigman, M., 187, 188
Simenson, R. J., 81
Simmons, J. E., 54
Simon, T., 94
Slosson, R. L., 192
Slosson Intelligence Test, 192–193
  scoring, 193
Smashed Window Picture, 149

Smith, A., 129
Social behavior screening, 196–199
Soft signs, 39–50. *See also* Developmental soft signs; Soft signs of abnormality
  detection, 43
  developmental, *see* Developmental soft signs
  interpretation, 41, 42
  and learning disabled, 43
  measurement, 41
  and psychiatric disorders, 42
  standardized evaluation, 48–50
Soft signs of abnormality, 46–48
  astereognosis, 46
  dysarthia, 47
  motor signs, 47. *See also specific types of motor signs*
  word-finding difficulty, 47
Sparrow, S. S., 198
Specialist, choosing, 4–5
Specific Developmental Disorder Not Otherwise Specified (NOS), 38
Speech dysfluencies, 134
Speech pathology, 133
Speech Perception Test, 180
Speech Sounds Perception Test, 147
Spreen, O., 135, 136, 143, 149
Springer, S. P., 96, 98
Stamm, J. S., 36
Standard Progressive Matrices, 116
Stanford-Binet Intelligence Scale, 195, 196
Stanford-Binet Intelligence Scale subtests,
  Birthday Party Picture, 149
  Delayed Response Test, 164
  Naming Object from Memory Test, 164
  Picture Vocabulary, 97

Stanford-Binet Intelligence Test, 13, 90, 148, 158
Stanford-Binet Intelligence Test-Revised, 191
Sterling, H. M., 191
Sterling, P. J., 191
Sterne, D. M., 165
Stone, C. P., 159
Stone, M. H., 165
Street, R. F., 94
Stress, 27, 34
  in the home, 68
Stroop, J. R., 124, 182
Stroop Color, 182
Stroop Test, 124–125
  scoring, 125
Subcortical dysfunction, 67
Sudden infant death, 42
Suppression, 46
Sutherland, J., 81
Suttell, B. J., 112
Sweeney, J., 188
Sweet, J. J., 181, 183
Synkinesia, 43, 44

Tactile Finger Recognition test, 123–124
Tactile Form Recognition Test, 124
Tactile function assessment, 121–124
Tactile memory assessment, 171–173
Tactile Performance Test, 171–173
  scoring, 173
Talley, J. L., 158
Tanguay, P., 187, 188
Taylor, H. G., 184
Teeter, P. A., 109, 126
Telzrow, C. F., 97, 193, 197
Terman, L. M., 148, 149
Test of Facial Recognition, 108
Test of Motor Impersistance, 45

Teuber, H. L., 104
Thorndike, R. L., 157, 195
Tic disorders, 28
Token Test, 141, 143–146
  commands, 144–145
  scoring, 144
Tolor, A., 115
Tourette syndrome, 27
  characteristics, 27, 28
  diagnosis, 28
  symptoms, 28. *See also* Tic disorders
  treatment, 28
Tourk, L. M., 131
Touwen, B. C. L., 40
Trail Making Test, 108, 109, 181, 182
  samples, 109
  scores, 110
Tramontana, M. G., 188, 189
Tremors, 47
Tuokko, H., 135, 136
Tupper, D. E., 40, 135, 136, 185
Turner's syndrome, 16–17
  profile, 16
  treatment, 16–17
Tzavaras, A., 108

Van Allen, M. W., 108
Vaughan, H. G., 131
Verbal fluency assessment, 148–149
Verbal memory assessment, 155–162
Vignolo, L. A., 141, 147
Vineland Adaptive Behavior Scales, The, 198, 199
Vineland Social Maturity Scale, 198
  See also Vineland Adaptive Behavior Scales
Visual agnosia, 87
Visual function assessment, 105–106

Visual impairment,
  hemianopia, 20
  lateral conjugate gaze, 20
  nystagmus, 20
  occipital lobes, 20
  quandrantonopia, 20
  scotoma, 20
  strabismus, 20
  visual agnosia, 20–21
Visual memory assessment, 162–171
Visual recognition, 106–107
Visual suppression, assessment, 123

Waber, D. P., 170, 171
Warrington, E. K., 107
Wasserstein, J., 94
Watson, B., 188
Wechsler, D., 80, 95, 116, 129, 154, 156, 159, 182
Wechsler Intelligence Scale for Children-Revised (WISC-R), xii, 10, 13, 80, 90, 91, 102, 146, 188, 195, 196
  deficits, 86–89
  history of, 80
  verbal *vs.* performance IQ scores, 81–83
Wechsler Intelligence Scale for Children-Revised subtests, 9, 80, 83
  Animal House, 182
  Arithmetic, 83, 84, 87, 154, 188
  Block Design, 83, 85, 88, 116
  Coding, 86, 88, 182
  Comprehension, 83, 84, 86, 154, 188
  deficit assessment, 84, 85, 86
  Digit Span, 74, 83, 84, 87, 94, 156–157, 160
  influences on results, 83–89
  Information, 84, 86, 154, 188

Mazes, 86, 129
Object Assembly, 83, 85, 88, 188
Picture Arrangement, 83, 85, 87, 96
Picture Completion, 85, 87, 188
Similarities, 79, 83, 84, 86, 188
Vocabulary, 83, 84, 86
Wechsler Memory Scale, 78, 159
  Logical Memory, 182
  Visual Reproduction, 182
Wechsler Preschool and Primary Scale of Intelligence (WPPSI) subtests,
  Block Design, 116
  Sentences, 159
Wedding, D., 73, 110, 121
Weikart, D. P., 190
Weinberg, J., 94
Weintraub, S., 148
Weiss, E., 94
Wells, F. L., 149
Wells, K. C., 36
Wepman, J. H., 138, 182
Werner, E. E., 191
Wertheimer, M., 110
Whitaker, H. A., 137

Wide Range Achievement Test-Revised (WRAT-R), 152–153
Wide Range Achievement Test-Revised (WRAT-R) subtests,
  Arithmetic, 153
  Reading, 98, 153
  Spelling, 153
Wilkening, G. N., 104, 105
Wilkes, N., 161
Wilkinson, G. S., 98, 152
Williams, D. T., 28
Wilson, B. C., 143, 160
Wilson, J. J., 131
Windmiller, M., 197
Wirt, R. D., 60
Wisconsin Card Sorting Test (WCST), 126–127
Wolfson, D., 109
Woodcock, R. W., 121
Workman, E. A., 195
Word Naming, 148
Word Test, 182
Wright, B. D., 165
Wright, F., 81
Wysocki, J. J., 181, 183
Wysocki and Sweet Screening Battery, 181–184, 185

SCREENING CHILDREN
FOR
BRAIN IMPAIRMENT

Richard Berg, Ph.D., was trained in clinical neuropsychology at the University of Houston and completed a postdoctoral fellowship in neuropsychology at the University of Nebraska Medical Center. Dr. Berg formerly worked at the St. Jude Children's Research Hospital in Memphis and currently directs the neuropsychology laboratory for the West Virginia University Medical Center in Charleston.

Michael Franzen, Ph.D., was trained in clinical psychology at Southern Illinois University and completed a clinical internship and a postdoctoral year of training in clinical neuropsychology at the University of Nebraska Medical Center. Dr. Franzen is currently Director of Neuropsychology for the West Virginia University School of Medicine in Morgantown and he serves as Director of Psychological Training and Research at Allegheny General Hospital in Pittsburgh.

Both of the authors have published widely in the field of clinical neuropsychology and are actively involved in ongoing research.

SCREENING CHILDREN FOR BRAIN IMPAIRMENT

Michael Franzen, Ph.D.
Richard Berg, Ph.D.

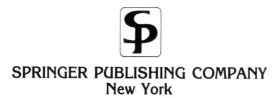

SPRINGER PUBLISHING COMPANY
New York

Copyright © 1989 by Springer Publishing Company, Inc.

All rights reserved

No part of this publication may be reproduced, stored in a retrieval system, or transmitted in any form or by any means, electronic, mechanical, photocopying, recording, or otherwise, without the prior permission of Springer Publishing Company, Inc.

Springer Publishing Company, Inc.
536 Broadway
New York, NY 10012

89 90 91 92 93 / 5 4 3 2 1

Library or Congress Cataloging-in-Publication Data

Franzen, Michael D., 1954–
    Screening Children for brain impairment.

    Bibliography: p.
    Includes index.
    1. Brain damage—Diagnosis. 2. Brain—damaged children—Medical examinations. 3. Pediatric neurology.
I. Berg, Richard (Richard A.) II. Title.
RJ496.B7F73   1989   618.92'80475   88-32742
ISBN 0-8261-6390-4

Printed in the United States of America

Contents

Introduction ix

Part I Cerebral Disorders in Children and the Specialists Who Treat Them 1

1 The Differing Roles of Professional Specialties 3
  Pediatrician 5
  Behavioral Pediatrician 6
  Pediatric Neurologist 6
  Child Psychiatrist 7
  Child Neuropsychologist 7
  School Psychologist 8
  Relationship Between Results of Neuropsychological and
    Achievement Assessment 8
  Overview 11

2 Developmental Disorders 12
  Mental Retardation 13
  Genetic Disorders 15
  Exposure to Neurotoxins 17
  Vitamin and Other Nutritional Deficiencies 18
  Sensory Disorders 20
  Auditory Disorders 21
  Language Disorders 21
  Overview 22

3 Neurological Disorders of Childhood 23
  Seizure Disorders 23

Hydrocephalus	26
Tourette Syndrome	27
Muscular Dystrophies	28
Other Disorders of Neuromuscular Development	29
Cerebral Palsy	30
Head Injury	30
Overview	32

4 Psychiatric and Behavioral Disorders of Children   33
Conduct Disorders	34
Childhood Schizophrenia	34
Affective Disorders	34
Anxiety Disorders	35
Eating Disorders	35
Infantile Autism	35
Attention Deficit Disorder	36
Developmental Motor Disorders	37
Learning Disorders	37
Disorders Not Otherwise Specified (NOS)	38

5 Neurological Soft Signs   39
The Controversy Related to Soft Signs	40
Relationship of Soft Signs to Neurological Disorders	41
Disorders Associated with Soft Signs	42
Classification and Assessment of Soft Signs	43
Neurological Dysfunction of Children (NDOC)	48
Physical and Neurological Examination for Soft Signs	49
Overview	50

Part II Evaluating the Child   51

6 The Interview and History   53
Interviewing the Child	53
Interviewing the Parents	58
Interviewing School Personnel	59
Obtaining the History	60
Conclusions	68

7 The Mental Status Exam in Children   70
Essentials of the Extended Mental Status Exam for Children	72
Attention	73
Language	74
Memory	77
Constructional Abilities	78
Higher Cognitive Functions	79
Summary	79

Contents   vii

8 The Wechsler Intelligence Scale for Children-Revised as a Screening Device   80
  WISC-R Verbal-Performance Discrepancies   81
  Wechsler Subtests as Screening Devices   83
  Effects of Brain Dysfunction on WISC-R Performance   86

9 The Kaufman Assessment Battery for Children   90
  Theoretical Basis of the K-ABC   90
  The K-ABC Subtests   92
  The K-ABC as a Screening Instrument for Brain Dysfunction   99

Part III Assessment Instruments and Their Uses   101

10 Screening Tests for Perceptual, Cognitive, and Motor Functioning   103
  Visual Functions   105
  Visual Recognition   106
  Complex Visual Functions   108
  Auditory Functions   118
  Tactile Functions   121
  General Cognitive Functions   124
  Manual Motor Functioning   129

11 Verbal Screening Instruments   133
  "Normal" Language Development   134
  Language Disorders in Children   135
  Childhood Aphasia   136
  Tests for Aphasia   138
  Screening for Verbal Fluency   148
  Academic Skills   150

12 Screening Children for Memory Functions   154
  Verbal Memory and Learning Problems   155
  Visual Memory Functioning   162
  Tactile Memory—The Tactual Performance Test   171

Part IV Special Considerations in Assessment   175

13 Screening Batteries for Children   177
  Screening Batteries versus Single Tests versus Comprehensive Test Batteries   177
  Wysocki and Sweet Screening Battery   181
  Florida Kindergarten Screening Battery   184
  The McCarthy Screening Test   185
  Screening Test for the Luria–Nebraska Neuropsychological Battery   186
  The Clinical Neuropsychological Evaluation Instrument   187
  Discriminant Equation for Screening for Neuropsychological Abnormality   188

14 Assessment of Very Young Children — 190
General Screening Devices of Cognitive Abilities — 191
Screening for Social and Adaptive Behavior — 196

Appendices
Appendix A Sample Interview Form — 203
Appendix B Common Tests Used in the Assessment of School-Aged Children — 208
Appendix C Common Tests Used in the Assessment of Preschool-Aged Children — 211
Appendix D Test Publisher Addresses — 213

Glossary — 215

References — 227

Index — 239

Introduction

This book arose partly out of the response to our earlier book *Screening for Brain Impairment* (Berg, Franzen, & Wedding; 1987). That book attempted to provide general clinicians working with an adult population with the basic knowledge to recognize and screen for the presence of organic etiologies. We decided to limit the information to adult disorders in order to maintain a reasonable length for the book. The response to that book has been gratifying and has influenced the decision to write the present one.

This book is intended for the general clinician who sees children as part of his/her professional practice. Often in the course of general practice, the psychologist or physician is asked to evaluate a child and determine whether or not an organic impairment is responsible for particular behavioral manifestations. Due to the limitations of training or experience, the general child clinician cannot be expected to provide a specialized assessment. However, they are still faced with the question of when to refer for a more extensive specialized evaluation which can be expensive in terms of time and money. This book is not meant to teach specialized evaluation; only years of didactic and experiential training can do that. But this book can be helpful in learning to perform an initial evaluation that can answer the question of whether to refer.

General child clinicians have already received specialized training in the area of child or pediatric practice. Optimally, this has included training in developmental theory. Just as this training sets them apart from adult general clinicians, so have child neuropsychologists received training that sets them apart from adult neuropsychologists. It is to a child neuropsychologist (or pediatrician, child psychiatrist, or pediatric neurologist as described in the first chapter of this book) that the child patient should be referred.

In an ideal world, the child patient has equal access to a wide variety of specialists. In the real world, access is limited due to geography and the limited amount of training experiences and institutions available to the professional seeking to become a specialist. Therefore, access to a specialist often involves extra effort and time as well as the additional distance required. Another consideration is the fact that parents or school teachers usually do not have the acumen required to recognize organic etiologies resulting in the referral of children with central nervous system etiologies to general child clinicians. They, then, must be able to recognize the possibility of an organic etiology and refer accordingly.

To evaluate the possibility of organic etiologies, it is necessary for child clinicians to utilize procedures that may not have been taught to them during their training. A major purpose of this book is to describe those procedures that can be employed without the additional specialized training of a child clinical neuropsychologist. Most of the procedures and tests described in this book can be acquired and used without a large monetary investment. Another purpose of this book is to educate the general child clinician as to the various type of disorders and their clinical presentations. A third purpose is to demystify the language and procedures of the child clinical neuropsychologist to further communication between the generalist and the specialist, thereby favorably effecting the overall level of patient care. For that reason, we have included a glossary of common technical terms. Finally, our experience with referring clinicians as well as our experience in developing curriculum and providing graduate education has indicated that most training programs do not currently provide adequate training in techniques to recognize and evaluate neuropsychological disorders. We hope that this book will be used in the training of future child clinicians to remediate that unfortunate but understandable problem.

We will not cover developmental aspects of behavioral and cognitive growth and change in this book. This is a very complex topic, and we do not feel we can do justice to the topic in the limited span of this book. By not discussing developmental theory, we do not mean to imply that it is unimportant. It is essential that every clinician who sees children has a working knowledge of developmental theory. In addition, the clinician should have knowledge of neurological developmental theory. There are many texts available, several of which are excellent. We would recommend Illington (1980, 1982). Failure to meet milestones at the usual time does not necessarily mean that the child is neurologically impaired, but it does raise the likelihood that a more complete evaluation might be in order.

Not every patient should receive every procedure described in this book. However, by studying this book the clinician can develop an outline for a

Introduction

child evaluation that seeks to uncover organic etiologies and aid in the decision to refer. The first step is to obtain as complete a history as is possible. The history may help to uncover organic etiologies as well as provide useful information to the specialist when the referral is made. If the history uncovers the possibility of an organic etiology, that particular problem area should receive special attention during the second step of the evaluation, the mental status exam. Finally, if the clinician judges herself to be competent in the use of the screening tests described in this book, those procedures can be administered in a further evaluation of the problem area. In no case are the procedures described in this book intended to take the place of an extensive specialized evaluation.

There are three possible outcomes of the extended mental status exam described in this book. First the evaluation may result in no indication of an organic etiology, in which case no referral is made. (Of course if there is any doubt, further evaluation is necessary to rule out the possibility.) Second, the mental status exam may result in a suspicion that organic impairment is present, in which case the child clinician performs one of the techniques described in the chapters on screening tests. This will allow greater specification of the type and degree of impairment present. Third, there may be sufficient evidence from the history and mental status exam to justify referral to a specialist.

In addition to the information contained in this book, clinicians can obtain information from the specialists to whom they may refer a patient. In general, we recommend that a consumer-oriented attitude be adopted by the clinician. Contact the specialist by telephone and describe the problem, asking for advice about whether a referral is warranted. Following referral and receipt of a report from the specialist, the generalist can again contact the specialist to ask for clarification and to give feedback about the usefulness of the report. Specialists tend to use jargon, and additional communication can avoid misunderstandings. Finally, the generalist can seek out a specialist with whom she feels comfortable and with whom a good pattern of communication can be developed. The specialist can provide feedback about the degree of specificity desired in the referral question, further increasing the quality of communication.

OVERVIEW OF THE BOOK

It would be impossible to contain in a single book all of the information necessary to evaluate a child and to screen for the possibility of organic involvement in the factors responsible for the child's behavior. It is even more apparent that it would be impossible to communicate the skills necessary to such an evaluation via the printed word. We therefore hope that clinicians and students who use this book will supplement it with additional readings and with supervised clinical experience. However, we feel that the information contained in this book cannot be found in a single source elsewhere. As mentioned earlier, in this book, we assume that the reader is familiar with the basics of child developmental theory, especially as it pertains to neurological and psychological aspects of development. We also assume that the reader is familiar with psychological assessment and with the clinical method.

The book opens with a discussion of the various roles of the different professionals who have chosen to evaluate and treat children. We hope this information will provide a basis for enhanced interdisciplinary communication and encourage each to use the other's skills to the benefit of the child patient.

The next section of the book gives an overview of some of the most commonly seen neurological and psychiatric/behavioral disorders in children. This serves to alert clinicians to the types of disorders seen and the common presentations of these disorders. Of course before treating children with these problems, more information is needed.

The following section presents aspects of the evaluation of the child that can be conducted without any special equipment and with the skills already in the possession of adequately trained child clinicians. These evaluative instruments are the interview, history, mental status exam, and the evaluation for soft neurological signs. Although most adequately trained child clinicians should be able to use these instruments, and may in fact be already using them, it will take a slightly different focus to implement the instruments as screening devices for organic impairment. The clinician can be guided here by the material in this book and by other knowledge obtained from the current literature and neuropsychologically oriented texts.

The next section contains several chapters devoted to specific assessment instruments. Some, such as the Wechsler Intelligence Scale for Children-Revised, are quite well known to most child clinicians. Others such as the Kaufman Assessment Battery for Children may be novel to the general child clinician because of their relatively recent appearance. Still other instruments, such as the Rey Auditory Verbal Learning Test, may be unfamiliar to the general child clinician because it has previously been used mainly in specialized settings.

The final two chapters are on topics that are not easily categorized with the previous chapters. There is a chapter devoted to a discussion of various screening batteries for children that have been suggested in the literature. The other chapter is a discussion of issues related to the evaluation of the very young child. Finally, the Appendices contain a sample interview form that readers can adopt and change to suit their own clinical settings and

Introduction

populations, a list of tests commonly used to evaluate school-aged children, a list of tests commonly used to evaluate preschool-aged children, and a list of test publisher addresses.

We hope that this book will be useful to the practicing general child clinician. We also hope that it will be useful to the graduate student. Both groups of people can use the book to increase their knowledge of cortical dysfunction and to increase their repertoire of clinical assessment techniques. Our ultimate hope is that the use of this book will help increase the standard of care for patients.

Alliant International University
Los Angeles Campus Library
1000 South Fremont Ave., Unit 5
Alhambra, CA 91803